CW00454909

Trust me, I'm a nurse...

Moira McGregor

Trust me, I'm a nurse...

A mid-life journey
from clerical to clinical

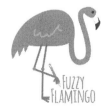

FUZZY
FLAMINGO

For Danielle and Kimberley
Whose support and belief in my ability to
do it all never waivered

For Bob
With love and thanks

For my beloved grandchildren

Contents

"Let us never consider ourselves
finished nurses… we must be learning
all of our lives."
Florence Nightingale

Introduction

I come from a very working-class family. The youngest and only girl in a family of five, I was never encouraged or expected to aim high, just to "do my best". My mother had several part-time jobs, sometimes three at a time. She often worked as a carer (or auxiliary nurse as it was then) and worked hard for minimal wages. She encouraged me to learn shorthand and typing in the hope that I would gain work in an office environment, rather than factory or low-level hospital work as, like every other working-class mother I knew, she wanted what she deemed to be a better life for me.

So, after leaving school with one O level in English, I learned Pitman's shorthand and I was pretty rubbish at it. In fact, classes usually consisted of us surreptitiously looking up naughty words or learning how to scribe "I love you" whilst thinking about the latest crush, but I don't remember much else. I went to evening classes to learn touch typing. The keyboard was blank and the letters were on a large blackboard on the wall, so there was no option but to touch type, and I actually got quite good at it. I then managed to secure several jobs where my typing skills were applied and appreciated.

I toyed with the idea of nursing when I was eighteen and was accepted into a large teaching hospital in Glasgow. However, an opportunity came up for me to go and work the summer season in Torquay as a chambermaid and waitress, which at the time seemed very glamorous and fun. The summer job won out and it must be said it wasn't glamorous but it was definitely fun.

When the fun ended, I went back to the security of a desk and a job I knew well by this time.

Life moved on I stayed in admin roles, got married and had two beautiful daughters, and any ideas of trying again to be a nurse were unrealistic due to the financial implications of a minimal bursary and shift working whilst managing a family.

Fast forward many administration jobs, most of them actually in hospital settings, a divorce (not beheaded, survived) and grown children, and I made a decision that it was time to further investigate returning to my childhood passion of becoming a nurse.

I hope that you will enjoy this journey with me and take some encouragement that, when it comes to further education and passion, the learning pool does not have an age limit for entry.

Administration to Medication?

Most of my adult life has involved working in administration; fifteen of those years in a hospital setting. I've always loved the atmosphere of a hospital, the smells – at that time disinfectant and flowers – the sense that everyone is busy, the multicultural world that is so inclusive – there seemed to be staff from every corner of the world, all bringing ideas, beliefs and customs that I was so interested in – but mostly the diversity of patients and the camaraderie of the staff across all disciplines.

In January 2003, I was working as a Ward Clerk, which involved sitting at a desk in the middle of the ward, fielding calls, passing messages, arranging porters to take patients for investigations and generally ensuring results, notes, etc., were in the right place at the right time, a role I had been in for eight years. I decided, over a few sleepless nights, that I wanted to experience the more hands-on aspect of caring – quite a daunting thought at my time of life, a mid-life crisis, some may say.

As a ward clerk, there had been many times I had sat at my desk on the ward and thought, "I'm sure I could do that." Well, here was my chance to try.

I decided to apply to be a bank auxiliary (now a healthcare assistant) and was accepted. This involved working shifts on my days off from being a ward clerk, hedging my bets, you see, always keeping a plan B in mind.

Bank Induction Day
– Auxiliary Workshop

S itting in a class full of people, where every single one – with the exception of me – had been involved in some way directly caring for patients was quite daunting.

We had talks on infection control, manual handling, fire lectures, occupational health and resus training (*please God don't let anyone depend on me for this*, I soberly thought). I learned the protocol for collecting blood from the blood bank, how to make a bed (hospital corners) and how to take a temperature and blood pressure. Does this all seem pretty basic? Well, nothing at this stage was too basic for me.

Moving and manual handling taught the correct procedures for moving patients without lasting injury to me or them using various weird and wonderful contraptions, always remembering the moving and manual handling acronym of the time: TILE – Task, Individual, Load, Environment. The trouble is, after this study day you don't normally think about it whilst performing various backbreaking tasks. Most nurses have bad backs: fact.

At the end of this induction period, I was mentally exhausted from trying to take in so much information. I was excited, apprehensive, worried... all the above; could I cope with all this? I did find that, having worked in the hospital setting for so long, some things must have subconsciously rubbed off and I found myself thinking, *how do I know that?* Having said that, there was an overwhelming amount that I didn't know. Experience was going to be a great teacher. So, the plan was: get a taste of nursing, do a bit of studying (a VRQ – Vocationally Related Qualification – in Contributing to the Care Setting) and see how it goes.

What a plan. First nursing uniform obtained, first taster shift booked, first of many doubts about my choices acknowledged.

First Orientation Shift

From being someone who was normally confident in their work, I was suddenly reduced to a quivering wreck on my first shift on an emergency admissions unit. I felt like the proverbial fish out of water. As soon as I appeared on the department in my crisp new 'first day at school' uniform, I explained to anyone who would listen that this was my first venture into the fray, basically hoping that I would not be too much of a hindrance.

The emergency admissions unit (EAU) of the hospital I worked at accepted patients directly from A & E for further investigations. Those people cross every spectrum of health needs; surgical, medical, mental health, the desperately sick and the not so sick. It was a busy, fast-paced environment full of inspirational people who have to know a little bit about lots of conditions. The atmosphere in the department was one of efficiency and expectancy, everyone appearing to know what they were doing. Well, everyone apart from me that is. It was noisy, handbells ringing with patients wanting attention, machines bleeping keeping a close check on cardiac patients who required monitoring, phones ringing, sometimes with anxious relatives seeking reassurance, sometimes notifications of yet more admissions, in retrospect probably not the best ward for me to choose for my induction shift.

The staff were very good, and I was paired with another auxiliary – with a much more impressively worn uniform – to shadow and learn from. When a 'runner' was required, I was first in line to volunteer; I knew I could run but I had yet to prove I could nurse.

As the shift went on, I started to settle down a bit and take it all in. One patient who remains in my mind was a tetraplegic (paralysed in all limbs) gentleman who came in with some bladder problems; his wife – permanent carer and loving partner – was with him. I assisted him with toileting, using my newly gained knowledge of manual handling, and generally tried to make him more comfortable, at the same time chatting to him to find out a little bit of background information from him. Now chatting I can do very well; I still have the school report cards to testify to that. Towards the end of my shift, the gentleman was transferred to the ward where I still worked as a ward clerk. I said my goodbyes and thankfully and wearily changed for home. I was physically and mentally exhausted but felt slightly better about it all than I had at the beginning of my shift.

The next day, back in my 'real job', I was chatting to

the patient from the previous evening, explaining my change of uniform. He said I had put him at ease on admission and thought I would make a good nurse… me! I explained to him that it had been my first shift and his opinion meant a great deal to me. In fact, I would have asked for it in writing if it wasn't for the whole paralysis thing! Onwards and upwards…

First Shift in the Numbers
(Depended On!)

After a couple more supernumerary shifts (these shifts were a blessing, you were not counted in the required number of staff, the pressure was off and the learning opportunities great), I was now being counted in the ward numbers, which was scary. People were actually depending on me to share the workload and contribute to the team. *Help, where is my nice, safe desk?* Before I went to the ward, I was very apprehensive about my total lack of experience. It was predominately a cancer ward, and I didn't know how I would feel. There were only eighteen patients that day and a small percentage of them were day case patients, having treatment before returning home. Although some patients were obviously very ill, it was a nice calm, relaxed atmosphere. It was apparent that some of the patients were regular visitors to the ward and had built great relationships with the staff and each other; for people going through cancer treatments, I'm sure this must be comforting. Several patients were neutropenic (I initially thought this may have been a rare, tropical disease), which I soon discovered means having a reduced immunity due to chemotherapy treatment. As a result of this, these patients had to be treated very carefully with regard to barrier nursing, with my gloves, apron, etc., protecting them from me and not me from them. I learned to take a manual blood pressure, using any available and willing arm of the staff to practise on, listening for the 'blub blub' instead of relying on a machine. Thank goodness for machines, but sometimes we have become too dependent on them. I came away from the ward feeling differently, a little bit more skilled and hoping to go back one day. The great thing about bank nursing is that it gives you the opportunity to work in greatly diversified areas and the opportunity to hopefully see what area(s) would be preferred long term. I think there is definitely an inclination towards either surgical nursing or medical nursing. Time would tell my preferred discipline.

Surgery, Wounds and Drains (Does this Learning Curve Never End?)

My first encounter of operation sites, drains and people in a pre- and post-operative state. Again, that voice in my head was saying, "I don't do wounds, can I do wounds?" There is a definite difference between seeing it from the safety of an admin desk and actually participating in the care and recuperation of patients. *Had I not realised this?* Ten minutes into my shift, a patient died (didn't touch her, honest). I was working with another auxiliary and a trained nurse, who asked me, when the time was right, did I want to assist with the necessary tasks for the deceased person before she left the ward. The choice was mine, no pressure. I thought about running, applying for a job in a supermarket, leaving the country... but alas came to the realisation that dealing with death was going to be a part of my role and I should face it. I begged, pleaded and generally told any staff that would listen (bless them all) that if at any time I felt uncomfortable with the task then I could leave; what a wimp!! This care involved gently washing the patient and getting her ready to be moved from the ward. Carrying out this very personal and final element of care for someone is not a task that can be said to be enjoyable, but what I can say is that if it had been my mother, grandmother, loved one, I was happy that she was cared for with a gentle dignity in death that was hopefully shown to her in life. The fragility of life is a sobering thought. Another experience and yet another bit further along the curve.

Bags of Rosé and No Not Drinkable (Urology)

By now I was starting to feel more confident in my ability to perform everyday tasks, such as bed making and washing. The great thing about being an HCA is that there is time to wash patients and, whilst doing that, they will tell you all sorts of things that they don't reveal to the trained nurses or doctors as they feel they are too busy. I loved washing my patients, making them look fresh and cared for when their relatives visited and learning all about who they were outside of their hospital bed. What a privilege. I have in my years of nursing looked after one of the original Tiller Girls and one of the Dambusters. A knowledge of their past does make a difference to how that patient may be viewed, and I would always encourage family to bring in photographs for the staff to pin above the bed. It's a gentle reminder to everyone that this is not the stroke patient, the dementia patient or the UTI; everyone deserves that dignity.

As well as the morning routine, I was suddenly

faced with the more technical tasks of measuring and emptying catheter bags, ensuring irrigation charts were accurate with descriptions of urine that would not look out of place in a 'guide to good wine' book. For example, light amounts of blood are often described as 'rosé'.

A Night at the Theatre

I took my first patient to theatre with another auxiliary – phew! Well, give me time, I was still learning, you know. He was off to theatre for bladder surgery and understandably nervous (I wasn't sure who was the most nervous, though, him or me).

Going down to theatre when you don't know what is expected of you is really quite daunting, so I was glad of the observational experience on this occasion. I watched as my colleague deftly placed the ECG pads where required, the positioning explained to me as RED (right side of chest) AMBER (left side) and GREEN (left side measurement below axilla) – just remember traffic lights, I was told!

I had never seen a patient succumb to anaesthesia before and was quite shocked by how quickly it all happened – one second awake and then, in a very short time, unconscious. Apparently, the role of anaesthesia is to stop the nerves from passing signals to the brain and I think what I found challenging was the speed at which that patient came under the effects of it. The sights, sounds and smells were strange to me and, if I'm honest, I spent half the time hoping I wouldn't pass out before they told me I could go; that achievement alone makes me very proud.

They Had Me Back

Another shift on the urology ward and they hadn't requested not to have me… (not quite the same as requesting me, but I would take it!) Maybe I wasn't too bad at this nursing thing!

This was a good shift as I was becoming more confident in my ability to contribute to the team and, just as I was basking in this feeling of euphoria, I was asked to take a patient to theatre, alone, arghh!

Practically before I got through the doors of the anaesthetic room, I was explaining that this was my first time (again), at the same time as reassuring the patient that I knew exactly what I was doing and it was all just a doddle (as they say in Glasgow). Now, was that red, amber, green or green, amber, red – oh dear!!

The anaesthetist on duty must have been sent from heaven – he was understanding and patient to the extreme. The patient was having a spinal block and he explained, in great detail, to both myself and the patient, the procedure. My patient, bless her, was very aware of my naivety and, having undergone several operations, was a source of information to me. My role was to be face-to-face with her sitting on the edge of the trolley whilst the anaesthetist placed the needle into the required space around her spine. As you can imagine, this was a very delicate procedure and demanded complete focus on helping the patient stay absolutely still. I did what I do best, I talked quietly and reassuringly and again marvelled at the trust patients put in us to care for them. I was fascinated, less tense than my first time and I didn't want to faint... Result!

'Eau de Poo' (Care of the Elderly)

Still doing bank shifts, I tried to vary the specialities I was going to as I thought this would give me a better understanding and be good for decision making if there came a time to decide if this was what I wanted long term.

My shift on a medical ward started badly, continued badly and ended badly. Working a twelve-hour shift on a ward that has an epidemic of sickness and diarrhoea was not fun, smart or recommended, but a part of being a nurse. One of my poor patients, as well as having these problems, was totally confused due to dementia and so objected strongly to being cleaned up frequently through the night. There was 'poo' on the side rails, the bed, his locker, his face, his nails... my arms, my face, my uniform... are you getting the picture yet, albeit not a very pretty one? A whole new meaning to the phrase getting 'sh*t-faced'. After a shift consisting of mainly the above, I was physically exhausted and had a continuous smell in my nostrils that definitely would not make the

Chanel counter. Having total empathy with my poor, exhausted patients, I did hope that, on some level, this particular patient realised that I hadn't been single-handedly determined to wash him so much he would get hydrophobia or to deliberately disturb his much-deserved sleep. Oh, the glamour of it all!

My next bank shift was on the cardiac unit, which wasn't as scary as you think as all the patients, although being investigated for cardiac problems, appeared reasonably well, they were monitored and it was a calm ward with the nursing team very supportive of bank nurses and grateful for their added help, and then...

Cardiac Arrest

D one the theory, read the books, attended a study day, so I knew what to expect, right? Wrong. My first cardiac arrest happened in the early morning following a night duty on the cardiac ward. Cardiac arrests were not as common as you may think on this ward, as cardiac patients are well monitored, and problems detected early. However, one of the patients collapsed on his return from the toilet. He was dressed, ready to go home later in the day after having some treatment and had appeared well. Someone got the 'crash' trolley, which pretty much has everything in it you need to try and recover a patient who has arrested. There are cannulas for fluids to be given, intubation materials, drugs and a defibrillator to restart the heart. A call was put out to the emergency team. Every hospital had a crash team of very experienced medical professionals who, as well as doing their daily jobs, carry a bleep and attend every cardiac arrest in the hospital. They have advanced training in life support and are constantly up to date with practice.

They are heaven sent when an arrest happens. Trying to be useful in a sea of very experienced, very capable people, I connected the oxygen and altered the tubing, which hadn't been cut to size (a valuable lesson for the future). The crash team arrived within minutes and, although I had previous experience of death, it had, up until then, been very peaceful and dignified. I found it shocking to watch and, unfortunately, the team were unable to bring the patient back. I was in awe of the individuals who worked tirelessly trying to resuscitate the patient and in despair for his poor family left behind. They had expected him home that day and the shock they were about to receive was just unthinkable. Following the event, the ward staff made a point of asking me how I felt and answered any questions I had. This debrief is after any traumatic situation and a good manager will always ensure it is available to their staff. I hoped I would not be involved in many of these incidents but if I was to be, I hoped I could act with the same professionalism and compassion as I witnessed. I have to say, I went home and had a cry; it was a very sad shift.

Definite Tug on the Heartstrings

Over the last few bank shifts on the urology ward, I built up a rapport with a lovely Irish gentleman. This is another one of the privileges of being an HCA: no mountains of paperwork to get through and more time to spend with patients. He, unfortunately, had inoperable cancer and had a difficult time in coming to terms with his prognosis. Despite this, he was never complaining, always grateful for each little task and just anxious to get back home. We talked about many things in our time together; his life as a young man (an eye for the girls), his liking for the horses, his many winners and I'm sure some losers, although he touched less on them, and his fondness for a glass – or two – of Guinness. On my shift, things had at last come together and he was able to be discharged, first to stay with his daughter and then to his own beloved home. Walking round the ward in his smart shirt and tie, sports jacket at the ready, keeping a beady eye on the door for his daughter, he looked relaxed, happy and at peace with himself. We had a hug, said our goodbyes and off he went. I have always felt privileged to meet and care for people when they were at their most vulnerable. Sometimes it's difficult not to be able to 'fix it' and it's not always possible to remain emotionally detached. Tears? What tears? Must have been the onion soup for lunch!

A Gigolo in a Plaster Cast
(Orthopaedics)

As well as the sad times, there are many cases that cheer you up and cause a bit of a giggle. This patient was admitted to hospital after coming to the area on a footballing weekend with the lads. Unfortunately, Ronaldo or Beckham he was not; a broken ankle followed thirty minutes on the pitch. His dutiful wife called from two hundred miles away each morning to enquire about his health and to express her concern... followed by his equally dutiful girlfriend and this, combined with a stream of female visitors, allowed for a great deal of banter about 'how it will all end in tears'.

A definite case for discretion on the telephone being an important part of the job.

Important in Death as in Life
(General Medical)

In the process of carrying out morning care, myself and another member of staff were attending to an elderly gentleman brought in the previous night when he suddenly stopped breathing. Could it be that I was a jinx? A call went out yet again for the team to attend when he spontaneously started breathing again (was he unaware he was making me nervous?!). The team decided after consultation with family members that, should it happen again, they would not resuscitate due to his multiple health problems. This involved a DNAR form (do not attempt resuscitation), signed and dated. Contrary to some public feeling about this, it does not mean you leave that patient to die, it means you allow them to pass in a dignified manner with compassion and care never forgotten. In due course, he started to lose his battle for life and, having nothing actively to do, I held his hand and gave reassurance to him that he was not alone as he peacefully slipped away. It was a thought-provoking experience being the last person with him, but an experience that I felt privileged to have been part of. Nursing is such a special job; you see people when they are at their most vulnerable and they often tell you things that they have not entrusted to anyone else. I hoped that I would never forget this or take it for granted.

The End... the Beginning

Six months had passed since I went on to the nursing bank. I had finished my VRQ and felt that I could now go on to a ward in my healthcare assistant uniform and make a valuable contribution to the team. I had met some lovely people and gained so much experience and immense job satisfaction. I made a decision to take the plunge and leave administration to apply for posts as a healthcare assistant. It was a lower salary than I'd had and I did lots of sums to ensure that I could still support myself and my two daughters in the process of it, which was daunting, but they were incredibly supportive of the changes to the routine we would all face and proud of their old mum for embracing the change. Future plans included completing an NVQ3 in Care and, from there, who knew, but life seemed good, I was enjoying my new role and was glad I'd decided to make the change.

A Real Nurse?

Well, here I was having somehow managed to convince the interview panel to employ me on my first permanent contract as a healthcare assistant; no more desk job for me. But wait… That meant no backup plan, no plan B. What if I didn't like it on a permanent basis? Arghh! My first role as an HCA was in the endoscopy department and was different to ward nursing, but surely I would be able to transfer some of the skills I had learned, wouldn't I? Here I went again, thinking about the potential difficulties and challenges after I had jumped.

Endoscopy nurses, at that time, covered three areas: outpatient department, procedure and recovery rooms and sterilisation/scope care. In the genre of Des Lynham: areas to learn, three; experience of each, nil.

Thank the Lord for supernumerary (again) and, just as an afterthought, as if I didn't have enough to focus on, I had been accepted on the NVQ training programme. Intense study as well as working, looking after my family and what else… oh yes, sleep! I really needed some sleep and rest from an overactive brain! I sensed a definite mid-life crisis going on here.

First Week in Endoscopy Unit

Supernumerary for a settling-in period allowed me to go into the procedures to watch and learn without being in the allocated staff numbers (ah, back to no one depending on me for a while, phew!). We had ERCPs (Endoscopic retrograde cholangiopancreatography), colonoscopies, bronchoscopies, gastroscopies; in fact, if there was an 'oscopy' going on, I was there! During these procedures, I tried to blend into the background at the same time as getting a good view and looking as though I was meant to be there. I did a lot of smiling and nodding in the hope of being accepted in the room. There was and still is something totally amazing about seeing the inside of the human body on a television screen. Whether the scope was expertly being directed down the oesophagus or around the colon, what impressed me most was the fact that people could differentiate between areas; to my untrained eye, it all looked remarkably similar. I watched, I listened to talk of lumens, ascending, descending and transverse (which incidentally looks like a Toblerone shape!) colons on one procedure and oesophagitis and reflux on the other. The method of applying torque – a twisting movement of the scope and not a 'posh' pronunciation of talk – was just another thing learned. I was thoroughly enjoying myself.

Scope Care

'd had my induction into the world of scope care, the internal workings, the lights, channels, air/water/ biopsy, umbilical, coherent and non-coherent fibre bundles. Confused? Me too! Brush each channel three times, not two, not four, but a definite three. Wash, flush, brush, rinse – and all this before the scopes are placed in the sterilisation unit. Then there was the handling of the 'snake-like' contraption, it must be coiled no smaller than a dinner plate or the fibres could be damaged. Well, are we talking 'Hungry Horse' dinner plates or Marco Pierre White dinner plates? You laugh, but it made a difference. These scopes cost an absolute fortune, so it was with trepidation I handled them, hoping that I was not going to be the one to drop it. Not sufficient to grapple it into a neat coil (of the correct size), I then had to stretch it out after cleaning to emit excess water. I have short arms. Oh, how it should have been part of the job specifications that long arms and the ability to judge a dinner plate size were advantageous. I failed dramatically on both counts, but I was there for the long haul, so I would learn – my children did wonder why all their belts and scarves were sorted into coils, dinner plate size, of course.

A Few Weeks and a Few 'Did I Do the Right Thing?' Moments On

was getting into the swing of it all now. I would go to work and change into my scrubs, feeling just like George Clooney's love interest in ER (well, no harm in dreaming). I could coil, I could clean and I could take patient observations, take cannulas out, drinks made, relatives contacted and off they went, none the worse for having had me to look after them. So, I was conquering this whole caring thing, but I wanted more. I was so inquisitive I wanted to know why one person had a disease and not someone else; was there genetics involved, or lifestyle choices, or both? I wanted to know the effects of drugs and the holistic effect on patients of illness. I had always been a 'people' person and I felt that I had a natural empathy and affinity for people, so in for a penny, in for a pound, I started to think about how I could train to be a registered nurse without bankrupting myself, keep paying my mortgage and maintain some sort of standard of living. The Open University had recently developed a programme designed to support workers to become registered nurses while still working on the job, which widened access to higher education for people just like me who could not afford to live on a minimal bursary but retain a salary whilst training. I applied for a place on the Open University nurse training programme training to become a registered nurse. I would say, like Pinocchio, I wanted to be a 'real' nurse, but that would take away from all the wonderful care assistants out there. I just wanted something more for myself and I suppose to prove to myself I could do it. As a Glasgow girl from a working-class background, university was never mentioned or encouraged as a post-school option, so this was a very big deal for me, but feeling I had something to prove, I terrified myself yet again.

First Day in Out-patients Surgical Clinic (Unimpressed Surgeon)

Well, this wiped the smugness from my face; a whole new setup to learn. I had a list (note: always have a list!) on how to set up trolleys for clinic. Bronchoscopes, flexis-sigs, swabs, KY, gloves, light source (source not sabre, *Star Wars* it isn't). My first clinic alone after shadowing for a time was with a surgeon – who, for professional, grovelling reasons, shall only be referred to as Mr P – and I fumbled my way through it. I passed the required instruments, perhaps not as quickly as he preferred; so many sighs can't be good for a person, and all that eye rolling! Now, where does that light source connect to? Meanwhile, I was reassuring the patient, encouraging relaxation while I was looking at a long, rigid, very rigid tube holding the appearance of an instrument of supreme torture and being very grateful that I was the one in the upright position. Clinic over, butterflies just about quelled and no disasters, phew! I don't think the patient realised my inexperience, but the surgeon… well, he just may have.

Open University Nurse Training

Applied and was rejected! Yes, you heard right, rejected, didn't even get an interview. In retrospect, I had not started my NVQ training yet, and I still had so much to learn, so maybe, just maybe mind you, they made the right decision; it sure didn't feel like it, though. I felt really disappointed and thought that maybe my role as a healthcare assistant should be enough. A very deserving colleague of mine got a place, so I was happy about that and, as they say, better luck next time, IF there was a next time.

NVQ Training

I was accepted to commence my NVQ3 training at the beginning of 2004 and hoped to complete it within the year. I thought that I may live to regret saying that, but a girl needs to have a plan, right? I had two great facilitators, Di and Julie, who I plagued the life out of to mark each component of it quickly to allow me to move on. I'm sure they dreaded my many calls to them. I had a mentor who was a highly qualified staff nurse in the endoscopy department, whose role was to coax, push and stretch me to enable me to complete all the components of the NVQ3 as quickly as possible, as I still wanted that OU place. I had the enthusiasm, Debbie had the red pen, what a team.

Talking – Now Here Is Something I Know How to Do!

Short staffing in the unit meant I was asked by Sister to come into the procedure and sit with the patient, do observations and offer reassurance; apologies to everyone I trampled over in the rush to get there! Offer reassurance? I did what I do best and talked to the patient throughout the procedure and talked and talked… not sure about her post-procedure pain, but her ears must have been on fire! She seemed pleased by the distraction, but perhaps she just said that to make me stop! Later, in the corridor, the consultant stopped me and said, "Well done, Moira, you were really good in there." *Moira?* I didn't even know she knew my name! I went home on an absolute high.

From a Learning Curve to a Complete Rotation

The unit was looking for staff, trained and untrained, to take part in a gastro rotation involving spending four months on a colorectal (lower GI) and four months on an upper GI ward. I felt I was just getting to know my colleagues and had so much to learn, but it would be a great experience for me to build up my skills. Okay, that's it, talked myself into it, again! I'm not sure what it was that made me think I could do everything, but after every decision, I definitely had a wobble and thought I should probably stop doing it.

Clueless Yet Again
(First Rotation)

On the first day of the rotation on the colorectal ward, there I was for four months on a ward dealing with major bowel surgery and I had never seen a stoma (colostomy), of which there are many. Some were temporary to allow the bowel to rest after surgery, and some permanent, when it is not possible to rejoin the bowel for various reasons. A colostomy involves bringing part of the bowel out through the abdominal wall and attaching a bag to collect waste. I had a 'fear of the unknown' feeling, and I was seriously doubting my decision to rotate. However, for the first two weeks, I was assigned to a 'buddy' to shadow and learn from; ah, that's better. On my first day, my buddy, a very informative and capable healthcare assistant, invited me into a side room to observe her carrying out a dressing. The patient was a young, teenage lad with a history of Crohn's disease resulting in an operation to remove the affected part of his colon and function a colostomy. Here we were then, my first experience of seeing a stoma. Not being enough, my buddy took the dressing off to see that the wound had de-hissed (a process where the wound breaks down and opens up). My first thought was *I feel faint*, my second was *does it show in my face* and my third *take deep breaths, look out of the window!* Sneaking the occasional glance and trying to focus on the patient, I managed to get through this first experience. I will admit that I struggled with coming face-to-face with what I viewed at that time as pretty brutal looking surgery. I felt ashamed of my reaction and actually doubted my ability to go on with nursing if this was how I felt when faced with a difficult situation. Nursing is all about what is called 'reflective practice': looking at how things were done, could you have done it better or differently and would the outcome have changed. It's also about reflection around your feelings, learning and growing, and is a really good skill to have in any walk of life. Reflecting on this particular experience when I went home, my initial reaction of *I can't do this* was replaced by *he has to cope with this all day, every day, get over yourself!* I felt very humbled.

Out and About

Part of my experience on the ward involved going out with the stoma nurse to patients in the community a few weeks later. I hoped that this would get me over my irrational fear of dealing with colostomies. After spending some time chatting about stoma care as a whole, we went on our first visit. Guess what! We visited the lad who had been in the side room. He was now at home self-caring for his stoma and wound. This time I watched him clean and care for the site and chatted to him about his feelings. He had several years of coping with pain and fatigue, missing out on teenage experiences, and he actually felt so much better having had the surgery. I didn't feel faint, I didn't need a window and felt very uplifted by my visit to a very nice young man. I have to say here that I remain eternally grateful to these trusting patients for their willingness to allow me to learn by experience.

Theatre Visit – Les Mis? Miss Saigon? Sadly No...

Being on a surgical ward, taking patients to theatre was routine. Remember my first time, red, amber, green? Old hat now! I loved accompanying the patients to theatre and reassuring them, but on this occasion, once the patient was asleep, instead of leaving, the anaesthetist, who remembered me from my days as a ward clerk (was that really in this lifetime?), was interested in how I was getting on and asked if I would like to assist in intubation. I completely ignored her as I thought she must be asking someone else but realised she WAS speaking to me. I was in there faster than a blink of an eye. She talked me through the positioning and supervised me throughout. What an amazing feeling; her faith and belief in me and her enthusiasm to impart her knowledge to me just reinforced for me that I was soooo in the right job. Thank you, you know who you are.

Another Theatre Experience

On one of my regular visits back to the endoscopy unit, I was lucky enough to be included in a team taking a patient to general theatre. The patient was to have a colonoscopy and a laparoscopy (a small opening in the abdomen to allow insertion of tools, usually either for diagnostic purposes or to do surgical procedures) done at the same time under general anaesthetic. This was my first experience of actually being in theatre during an operation and those old butterflies were back. The smells, the strict protocol to be followed and the number of staff around made me feel particularly useless and ill at ease. I made a mental note of exits, in case of fainting; be prepared and all that! I was very worried about touching anything in case I unwittingly contaminated a sterile area, so, once more, I blended into the background (I was getting quite good at it!). Once the procedure started, I was engrossed. Two television screens, one showing the scope travelling through the inside of the colon, and one showing a scope in the abdomen. At one point, the lights from both scopes reflected on each other and it was like a ghostly scene from the exorcist. I was loving my job!!!

Another Shift, Another Adventure

had built up a good relationship with a patient recovering from major bowel surgery. She was a registered nurse and sympathetic to my ongoing learning curve. One particular shift, she came out of the shower saying her stoma bag had burst and she needed help. Here I went with my thoughts again: *I must get a real nurse who knows what they are doing*, looking around, but alas there was only me. This poor patient was in the middle of a nightmare situation and was blessed with ME! Pulling her curtains and grabbing the nearest receptacle, I donned the latex and thought *here we go*. Considering that, not so long ago, I felt physically sick at the sight of a stoma, I was understandably a little nervous (understatement). My patient was amazing and talked me through the whole procedure (a slight role reversal, but it worked for both of us); she knew what to do but couldn't do it, I didn't know what to do but was willing to take instruction. Job done, we sat and had a chat. She opened up to me about her feelings of having a colostomy bag and how she dealt with it. It was such a privilege that she felt she could confide her feelings in me. Maybe I didn't carry out the task as quickly or as expertly as someone more experienced, but next time I wouldn't be thinking *get me a nurse*, I will be thinking, *stoma, no problem*!

Clip Happy

By now, I was doing dressings, getting my trolley ready, aseptic (non-touch) technique, check me out, sounding as if I know something! I was asked if I wanted to observe a patient having his wound clips removed. Of course, me being me, I refused nothing but blows. Watching the nurse remove them deftly and the wound looking great was fascinating. She asked me if I wanted to try. Did I want to try? I almost took her hand off snatching the clip removers! The patient very kindly consented to being my practice model, bless him, so off I went. My hand was shaking so much I felt I had to confirm for the patient that I wasn't in alcohol withdrawal, merely a little nervous in case I hurt him. Clip remover gently eased under staple, press down and with a gentle rocking motion the clip came free, there, done it! Patient still smiling, so I carried on, two, four, eight... I got to twenty-six and it was all over, oh no, I was on a roll! I didn't want to stop. I laughed and joked with the patient that I was going on the prowl looking for wounds to unclip.

Another Chapter

For the next part of my rotation, I had a new ward, a new buddy, for a time, and perhaps a new outlook. Patients on this ward included people with alcoholic liver disease and eating disorders, along with other gastrointestinal problems. The challenge there was for me to accept that we may get people over their acute episode only for them to self-discharge back to their life of alcohol dependence. I was not proud of the fact that I sometimes found it hard to sympathise with certain patients who came in demanding to be cleaned up, only to self-discharge when it suited. Could I adjust to this ward? Time would tell.

Perceptions

One patient on the ward, N, had been admitted with complications associated with suffering from a long-term eating disorder. On previous occasions, she had been sectioned under the Mental Health Act for treatment but, on this occasion, she was there freely. What can I say about N? She was a very introverted and sad girl with a host of emotional issues. She liked to go out for a cigarette and needed an escort, which sometimes was me. It was during these times that we built up a relationship, although it was strictly on her terms, and I sometimes felt very helpless when she tried to self-harm or induce vomiting. The background to N's life allowed a little insight into her behaviour and, while caring for her, I sometimes felt sympathy, sometimes despair, sometimes anger, not *at* her but *for* her. Mostly, I just tried to appreciate her multiple problems, both past and present, and hoped that one day she would find the strength to surmount them. It was very difficult for me to realise that I couldn't always make a difference.

Update

I was now halfway through my NVQ and I had applied for acceptance onto the nurse training programme for the second time. I did feel that I had a much better understanding of nursing and I had been pretty naive to think they should have taken me the first time I applied. I had grown and changed as a person, but my dream to be a qualified nurse had not diminished. Watch this space!

You Have to Laugh!

Another shift and one of my patients was admitted with various social and medical problems, one of which was alcohol-related dementia. The man was the same age as me and it saddened me to see what had become of him, but he was courteous and pleasant and we got on well. He couldn't remember me from one shift to the next but, on the upside, he was constantly meeting 'new people'! I will call him R. He had very long, infected nails, matted hair, a very bad skin condition and a general appearance of neglect. Assisting him with a much-needed shower one day, R asked me if I thought he was putting on a little weight. "You look fine," I replied.

"Oh good," said R, "I do like to look my best." Bless you, R, you put a smile on my face for a very long time. No one in my experience sets out to be an alcoholic or a drug addict. Everyone has a story and some of those stories make you realise that but for good fortune, that could be any one of us.

Interview for OU

Yeah! I am offered an interview this time for a place on the Open University course. My letter stated that I was expected to do a five-minute presentation on 'How I will change and how my role will change as a student nurse'. Five minutes is a long time to talk about yourself. I mean, I could talk for England, but not when something was so important to me. Eventually, I did a draft, got lots of people to read it and input suggestions and went off to the interview.

A panel of three asked me about prioritising care, what I perceived a good nurse to be, and various other questions, including 'what would you do if' scenarios. I wanted to say I would run at some but restrained myself. Anyway, I came to the five-minute talk and, taking into account nerves and my Scottish accent, which got faster and faster, the five minutes lasted about two. I heard a voice say I felt confident about the academic element to the role (it couldn't have been my voice because I knew I would definitely struggle!). I had to wait to find out, but I was not convinced my blagging skills were enough.

Back to My Friends and Colleagues, Hopefully Wiser

A s my rotational experienced finished, I was back in the endoscopy unit. I hadn't forgotten how to coil or how to be part of the unit team; thank goodness for that all-important coiling technique! It was nice to be back and hopefully I brought a newfound knowledge (and lots of anecdotes) with me.

Fanfare!

was driving the car and had a missed call from the hospital. I knew it could be the results of my interview, so I pulled the car over and tried to compose myself before ringing back. I was informed I had a place BUT it was dependent on passing a numeracy test, as I didn't have a GCSE in maths. *A little test*, I thought, *not too bad*. But no. I had to go – with others in the accepted group – to college for a total of ten weeks. twice a week for tutorials and then sit an exam at the end of it. I left school a very long time ago, and while I had always been okay with figures, I was feeling the pressure. I had a wobble and started to think that maybe my ambitions were a little beyond my capabilities. Maybe it just wasn't meant to be and passion would not be enough.

Chocolate and Numbers

The first night at maths class, I arrived from work, as did most of the others, and I was tired, hungry and disillusioned about the whole thing! I met the girls who, if we passed, would become close colleagues for the next four years. The class commenced. We were told about how to round numbers up – primary school stuff – and how to do percentages using chocolate bars to dissect! Did this woman not realise that I didn't care how many pieces the chocolate bar could be divided into? I was so hungry I WANT THE CHOCOLATE, GIVE ME THE CHOCOLATE!!! So many weeks to go, infinitely more difficult stuff to come, that wobble was getting more unstable by the day.

The Right Decision

When I went to work one day in the endoscopy unit, due to staff holidays and sickness, there was a trained member of staff short for a list. The nurse in charge had agreed that an HCA could cover, under supervision. *PICK ME, PICK ME...* I refrained from saying it out loud and tried to behave cool and professional when it was agreed for me to cover (as if!). My role was to admit the patients, stay with them during the procedures to monitor observations, getting responses from them and to pass on any relevant information to the team regarding pain or a change in condition. I was SO ready for this. To cut a very long story short (I am trying), I will only relate two patients. Whilst having the procedure done under sedation (the aim is to keep the patient aware but drowsy and calm), J told me all about his annual Caribbean cruise. He asked to watch the television monitor during the procedure and asked me what part of the colon they were at. Luckily, I recognised 'the Toblerone' and confidently answered:

TRUST ME, I'M A NURSE...

"The transverse colon." The team looked impressed. I didn't share that had he asked me at any other point in the procedure, I would not have had a clue; nice one, J.

My next patient was R, an elderly gentleman who had a bit of trouble during the procedure requiring increased oxygen and medication. After initial intervention, he remained stable; however, this event had tested my observational skills and my ability to stay calm. Yes, on the outside, maybe, but inside I had the old butterflies back and the excitement left me buzzing (was that wrong?!). The patient, I had to say, remained well.

The list went on all day and my enthusiasm never waned. I talked, looked, listened and absorbed it all. Is it wrong to wish your colleagues would go off sick and have holidays more often? Each time I experienced a situation where I could contribute, it only confirmed for me that the decision I made to go into nursing was the right one. My bank account wasn't seeing black ink, I got stressed and tired trying to do it all, but I could go home on a day like that day feeling on top of the world!

Carol Vorderman
Eat Your Heart Out

The day of the maths exam arrived, and I quickly realised that my fear of exam situations had not diminished. By the time I turned the paper over, my brain was struggling to remember 1+1=2. I answered to the best of my ability important questions like how many packs of fish fingers of a certain size could fit into your freezer drawer – I was never going to bulk buy fish fingers, so relating to this did not come easily. I came out feeling decidedly unsure of my abilities and, knowing how much depended on me passing, I felt ever so slightly sick.

Some Weeks Later

PASSED the maths test! That's it, I would start my training in a few months! I bought a chocolate bar to celebrate (but didn't dissect it!).

In the two years since I'd first decided that I would like to try my hand at nursing, I had completed a VRQ, an NVQ3, went back to school for certificates in literacy and numeracy and been accepted for nurse training. I would start the following week on a whole new path, which for the next four years would be filled with study, study and more study! I was proud of my achievements so far. I had enjoyed many positive experiences, some sad moments, some funny moments and all the time I had been supported by everyone, my children, my friends and my colleagues.

I looked in the mirror and I couldn't quite believe the person looking back at me had achieved all this in such a short time. Sadly, my mum was no longer around to see this, but I just know she would have been immensely proud of my achievements from afar.

As I embarked on this next stage of my life, I was

a little bit closer to reaching my goal. The saying 'it's never too late to learn' comes to mind! There was a part of me that still doubted my ability to make it as a registered nurse, but I would have a damn good try. Now what was it that great man said, "I had a dream"!

And So to Work!!

The excitement and anticipation of gaining a place had settled and I was in an anticlimax situation; still working as an HCA in endoscopy and just itching to get started on the next part of my journey.

All the books I required in the first three months of training had arrived and... panic... how would I ever understand all of this? There was one TMA (tutor marked assignment) to complete almost every month and just reading the titles brought me out in a cold sweat! Panic was setting in. I had no real academic achievements (not to dismiss my one O level), apart from my NVQ. My mother told me when I left school I should learn shorthand and typing and I would always get a job. To be fair it had stood me in good stead for many years but I was not sure I had the academic ability to complete this course. Friends said I was brave, but I was feeling very scared and vulnerable, thinking I had aimed a little bit too high! Okay, breathe, just breathe. I put the books away and prayed for inspiration.

Student Nurse McGregor!

I t was official, I'd become an Open University Student of Nursing (and I had another new shiny uniform to prove it!). Putting on my uniform for the first time, my feelings equated to having that much coveted designer outfit (albeit cheaper). I felt so proud to be wearing it. I had arrived – well, at least at the start of a long, steep learning curve, but I would give it my all and hope that the doubting Thomas sitting on my shoulder would do one!

I had met my cohort, some during the maths lessons and some for the first time; a varied mix of people from different backgrounds but all working as health care assistants and all with one aim in common. I was the eldest in the group, which worried me slightly, but I am pleased to say that was never an issue to our camaraderie and friendship. We all vowed to support each other during the course – and I am happy to say that support never wavered. We all had wobbles at one point or another, but it was great to be able to talk them over with people who understood. My daughters, who had either been or were in university at this time, were also a great source of positivity and help to me.

The Open University pre-registration nursing course is a work-based programme taken over four years. At that time, it involved continuous assessment, from TMAs (tutor marked assignments), witness statements from evidence-based practice, portfolio submissions and an examination, 306.5 days (2300 hours) of study and 253 days (1900 hours) of supernumerary practice on various placements. I thought a lie down in a darkened room may be in order!

The first year was purely theory, which meant that I would continue to work in Endoscopy, although now, as a student nurse, I had a trained nurse as a mentor. David was knowledgeable, supportive and accessible for all my concerns, which I was extremely grateful for (and as an afterthought he always smelled amazing!). I had study days to attend lectures and to revise for assignments, so I was working full time, running a home and studying. Was I concerned? You bet I was. But also very grateful that my Healthcare Trust had seen fit to invest time and money into my training and allow me an opportunity that I may not otherwise have been in a position to take. I had assessment guides, audio CDs, course website activities, a handbook, textbooks – I was feeling the panic setting in again – maybe I had actually punched above my weight this time; a definite case of imposter syndrome was nibbling away at me.

Academia

The first TMA, which consisted of an essay, evidence of competence in various settings and a multiple-choice sheet, was due in three weeks. Some of my group had been working on it for a few weeks and I had not started yet. My style of learning had been explored and I was deemed an 'activist' – apparently a doer not a thinker. My aim was to get myself into a routine where I did not leave everything to the last moment. I wanted to be the girl who had her essay prepared, proofread and typed at least two weeks in advance. Did I think this would happen? Hmmm!

The first-year essays or TMAs were mainly about understanding health and social care in general and the holistic needs of people. I met the fictitious Lynne and Arthur and became involved in their stories of being carers. I learned about institutional behaviour by studying the impact of Lennox Castle hospital, a castle built in the 1830s but converted in the early twentieth century into what became an infamous psychiatric hospital. Although initially hailed as being ahead of its time, it became vastly overcrowded, understaffed and underfunded. A study by the British Medical Journal in 1989 found that a quarter of all patients were dangerously underweight and malnourished, and cruel punishments and neglect also came to the forefront. The hospital finally closed in 2002, sending any remaining clients to reintegrate into the local community or to more modern psychiatric units. Part of my study was to watch a video of these people who shared their experience. This must have been so difficult, and the stress of these long-stay patients cannot even be imagined. It was heartbreaking. There was a gentleman who was adopted as a baby and later sent to Lennox Castle, but he never knew why. He never saw any family or friends again. People who were pregnant out of wedlock or stole a few pennies from a purse were abandoned as mentally ill to suffer all the inhumanities for many, many years, leaving them totally institutionalised and dependent.

I have to say, I was really enjoying the sociology part of the course and loved to understand how people thought and why herd immunity from vaccinations and illnesses is still a valid process, but would it make me a better nurse? I wasn't sure at this stage.

Now I have always thought I could write a reasonable essay; well, I did get O level English (I may have mentioned that before). However, I now had to learn a completely new style of writing, acknowledging plagiarism (when I was at school this was called copying) citing references using Harvard referencing; I felt like I had to learn a new language.

I read the desired material to help with my essay, A Healthy Community, but if someone had asked me five minutes later what I had read, I would not have a clue. Maybe it was menopausal brain? Maybe I was just too old to learn? Maybe I needed a glass of wine? The third maybe won the day…

Positive thinking ensued. I had read the units, listened to the tapes, embraced poverty and inequality and written the essay and posted it. Posting it was a problem, though. Suddenly my hands were stuck to the envelope as though they had superglue on them. The sweat, tears and immense support from colleagues and family it had taken to get this first TMA done had made me incredibly possessive of it.

Practice Practice Practice

Non study days were spent in the endoscopy unit. However, since becoming a student, I was now encouraged to learn more practical skills, and one day I was to develop my skills in using biopsy forceps during procedures. This involved the nurse (ta da!) handling the forceps and passing them down a scope. The consultant would then guide the nurse when to open/close the small, toothed area at the end to take a little piece of skin for biopsy purposes.

I had taken some out-of-date forceps home and practised a little. The apples in my fruit basket looked as though we had termites and my girls were afraid to sit still in case I pinched them, but this open and close business was becoming less scary. The patient was admitted into the room, the procedure was underway, and the doctor asked for biopsies to be taken. The fight or flight adrenaline kicked in and I definitely wanted to run for the hills, but I uncoiled, stretched and passed the forceps. Open/close and yes, I was there. Now I had to retract them without losing my precious piece of tissue. I must have looked as though I was fishing for the big one, arms outstretched, taking up more room than any one person is entitled to; how did the other nurses manage to make it look so effortless? Anyway, I placed my biopsy forceps in the biopsy pot, gave a little swirl and, oh yes, I had some tissue. "Let's take a few more," the doctor says… does he not realise how much concentration I have just used?!

My first TMA arrived back in the post. I wanted to open it, but I was so worried that I had dramatically failed. After realising that the results would not change no matter how long I stared at the envelope, I opened it… 63%… as 40% is a pass, you can understand why I was now dancing around the room in my underwear – never a pretty sight! No one was at home, so I had no one to tell. However, very soon the jungle drums kicked in and all my cohort had been contacted… we all passed, what a feeling! I must mention here that the comments were not all good and there was lots of red ink being bandied about and, apparently, I was "too chatty" in my text. In fact, I realised I had a very long way to go but one down, six to go for this year; onwards and upwards.

Procrastination

I had a study day. I had washed up, put a wash on, changed the beds, ironed... now, anyone who knows me will tell you I hate ironing with a passion, it is the most thankless, tiresome task, BUT it was better than studying. I was told it is called procrastination and I got the feeling I was going to become very familiar with it. When I finally got my head around it, I started taking notes. I had a difficult time relating some of the sociology to the patients I cared for, but I was beginning to understand the holistic idea. Doubting Thomas was still hanging on in there, although I was trying to shake him off once and for all.

My life seemed taken up with TMAs, tutorials, study days and work. I don't regret it for a minute, but it is incredibly hard work. I constantly stressed that I was too old to retain all this newfound knowledge and produce it at the right time. TMAs were coming back, and the marks were going in the right direction, so something must have been sinking in, after all. The TMAs were doing what they were meant to do, I think, and making me think about society as a whole. Part of me felt I just wanted to get on the wards and get on with it and the other part was scared stiff of doing just that.

My next TMA asked that I gave an argument for and against corporal punishment by parents. Every time I got an assignment through, my immediate thought was *I can't do this* followed quickly by *why did I ever think I could?* Now, I come from a background where, if I was misbehaving or being disrespectful, a clip round the ear was acceptable – not just by my parents, I hasten to add, but by any of the neighbours witnessing it! It's an emotive subject and subjective in its interpretation. What I can say is that I still remember being at school and being made to stand with my arms outstretched one hand on top of the other and a thick heavy leather belt coming into contact with my trembling hands. I was left with a face burning with embarrassment and hands burning with pain and heat. I cannot recall what I did to deserve this on either of the two occasions it happened, however I was not a particularly rebellious child and I still fail to understand why it seemed acceptable for a grown adult to subject a child to this. As they said in the learning outcomes… discuss.

Our cohort were always communicating with each other about how difficult days were or how to express on paper what we were thinking and each one of us at some point needed that someone a little more to encourage and support us. We had graduated into smaller groups of closer friends but still remained supportive of everyone. Thank heavens for my fellow students, wine and chocolate to get me through. I think I should give myself some health promotion information!

Work Days

My days at work looking after patients and not bending over books were still my preferred days and the day had come to be given my own list of patients in endoscopy. I admitted, assisted, recovered and discharged all my own patients without any disasters. What I found amazing, and still do, is that because I was in uniform, not so shiny and new now, patients automatically put their trust in you; what a huge responsibility.

The first year had gone very quickly and my marks appeared to be acceptable; in fact, I achieved an end of year portfolio distinction! I enjoyed my cohort learning days better than my self-led learning/procrastinating days.

I had started this course single but in the first year had met someone whom I thought could be special to me. Fortunately, he was understanding of my need to work and study and then work some more. He didn't live in the area, so a long-distance relationship seemed a good idea. I had time to study and work and then managed to fit a life in every other weekend. The programme followed the same general balance of study and ward placements as nurses going through the more conventional route. I was both apprehensive and excited to get notification of my first placement areas: orthopaedic and cardiac.

First Placement

My closest friend on the cohort was Tracy. She came from a primary care background and had never worked, nor had any desire to work in a hospital setting. Her aim was to become a practice nurse; however, she needed to complete the NMC requirements to gain registration and most of that was in a hospital setting. We had both been allocated orthopaedic wards for our first placements. Although different wards, I quite confidently thought I was going to be fine, but my work/study/wine buddy was terrified, and I think she would have run for the hills if she could. Promising to be there for each other, we both went off to start our first practical placement.

Now, the staff in endoscopy had known me as an HCA and supported my transition to a student nurse, actively seeking out experiences for me and imparting all their knowledge to me in the most supportive way. I suddenly felt as though I was on my own and had to prove to my new ward mentor that I was up to the challenge. My first day on orthopaedics was spent making beds, washing and answering bells. Disillusioned, I felt I was taking a step back, but decided not to rock the boat. I needed the staff on side to enable me to complete the placement and meet my knowledge criteria. Two weeks later, I was still making beds, washing, answering bells, and I decided I needed to speak to my mentor. I was told that I needed to learn the basics, despite being an HCA previously, and did I not realise this was the very basics of nursing? The HCAs on the ward, rather than being pleased that 'one of their own' was trying to learn whilst appreciating their role appeared to go out of their way to make my days difficult. I was not 'too posh to wash', but I had learned the techniques of bed baths, feeding, changing and toileting, so I had to emphasise that I had new skills to learn and that I needed her help to gain them. I made a decision to grab every opportunity in my supernumerary state and leave having developed as a person and a student nurse. I went to theatre to watch hips being replaced – amazing but appearing quite barbaric at times with hammers, chisels and a horrendous smell of surgical cement – constantly concerned about fainting yet again. Not my forte, I think. Tracy's ward manager and staff, however, were much more supportive, and I think she felt less concerned and disillusioned than me in the end.

My first placement never did get any better and I felt unsettled, wondering if I had made the right decision. But, as always, my fellow students, my course tutor and my overall mentor David picked me up, dusted me off and made me start again. One good thing about learning is that, as well as being inspired by very good nurses and managers, I learned what kind of nurse I did not want to be. Like in every other walk of life, there are nice people and not so nice people; nursing is no different. We are not all angels. In fact, if my halo slipped any more it may choke me! We are just human beings doing a job, sometimes not knowing when it's time to change direction.

Earning Whilst Learning

I n between working, studying and living, I decided to do some bank shifts in my local hospice. I thought it would give me an insight into another side of nursing (and my bank account needed to get out of the red) and did it ever. Hospice nurses are an amazing breed of people and the care they give to patients is second to none. It is a happy place. Yes people die there, but many more come in to have pain brought under control and to go back to spending some more quality time with their families. I learned so much about courage, strength and the will of people, and I also had some laughs.

One patient, I'll call him Jim, who had a terminal illness had been in and out of the hospice and had built a good relationship with the staff. I was on a night duty, and it was a very quiet and peaceful place at night. An old building, it could also possess an eerie quality about it. Jim was in a single room that led on to the garden and his bell rang around 2am. Entering the room, Jim was not in the bed and, after checking the toilet, was not there either. I was feeling confused and a little worried. I went further into the room to check the floor on the opposite side of the bed hoping with everything I had that he had not collapsed. As I got round, a figure appeared at the French doors and I almost passed out. Jim had put the sheet over his head and jumped out to scare me. He had decided to do his 'haunting' while alive to see how it would feel. Once my heart stopped racing, we had such a laugh about it.

I continued to do bank shifts in the hospice to supplement my meagre income and I witnessed hospice staff helping a young mother to make memory books for her two young children, parents watching young adult children die and agonising over something that is out of the natural order of things, and at the other end of the spectrum helping someone who has lived a full and happy life have a dignified and peaceful end. I consistently felt humbled by the strength of people facing the worst of situations and I think this experience went some way to affirming my 'glass half full' outlook on life.

I was still submitting my regular TMAs, written reflections and learning and evidencing basic skills. I recall thinking *well, I can take a blood pressure and temperature from my HCA days, so do I really need all this?* However, I quickly learned the difference was that I had to understand the mechanics of it, how the body temperature is controlled and what exactly systolic and diastolic blood pressure means. Again, I realised I had much to learn and a long way to go.

Another Place(ment),
Another Time

My second placement was on a urology ward, and I was back to rosé urine and bladder irrigation. I loved it. I used to work on this ward as a ward clerk and again had a supportive team in tow. My mentor, the ward sister, was someone I had become friends with previously. If I thought Gill was going to give me an easy time, I was soooo wrong! Every decision I took, she asked me to offer the rationale for it. She constantly pushed me and put me in situations that I would have to get comfortable with. She taught me about the value of a good handover from one shift to the next, concise but informative, and the value of carrying a notepad at all times. I learned and practised the art of catheter placement and removal (ouch!), the varying colours of acceptable urine and, in general, how to be a professional. I left that placement with more confidence in my abilities and our friendship also held out, so a good mentor can make a world of difference to a student nurse, and I vowed one day to become one. I just had to qualify as a nurse first!

Stay Safe Bus

I was then, and remained in the future, thirsty to learn and to enhance my skills, so any opportunity that came my way was gratefully, if naively, accepted. Torbay (where I had moved to when my children were little) had initiated a stay safe bus scheme, which was located by the harbour at the weekend between the hours of 9pm until 2am. This bus was akin to a minor injuries unit and was intended to keep people out of A & E. Everyone working on the bus was entirely voluntary and aiming to help anyone who needed it; the incoherent drunk who could not persuade a hard-working taxi driver to allow him to potentially vomit in their cab was given coffee and sympathy until sober enough to be put in a taxi; the girls who thought their drinks may have been spiked, which was hard to tell as they had already consumed a lot of alcohol – and the lost and stranded. I volunteered for quite some time and hopefully saved A & E a few visitors. I would be reminded of the poem etched in bronze onto the Statue of Liberty: "Give me your tired, your poor, your huddled masses". I just didn't really want the tired, poor masses vomiting on my shoes, but alas they did.

Theatre

Theatre placement next. Now, I loved the theatre – *Blood Brothers*, *Chicago*, *Les Mis* – what I wasn't so keen on was blood. What a scary place this was! The staff seem to be a breed apart and were a very insular lot. My first day there transported me back to the time I mentioned earlier when I took a patient to the anaesthetic room and felt faint. This time, however, I was expected to actually go into the theatre and watch. I had previously been to orthopaedic theatre to observe, but this time I was there for an eight-week placement and expected to gain quite a lot of knowledge in that time; head up, breathe in, Rescue Remedy on tap!

My first day, I was put in a surgical theatre to observe a hysterectomy. I felt physically ill, I had Rescue Remedy in my pocket and if anyone observed me occasionally (several times, really) open up to put drops on my tongue, they were too polite to mention it. The atmosphere of a surgical theatre is very strange. Everyone knows what their role is, there is the anaesthetist, ODP (operating department practitioner), surgeon, scrub nurse, runner, me... I was asked to move position to enable me to see better (*but I don't actually want to see*, I was thinking) and so I tried to look as cool as possible and move closer. I was warned (several times) to keep my hands by my side. DO NOT TOUCH ANYTHING! I was so worried about touching anything I had my hands behind my back holding on to each other for dear life. I hoped behind my mask no one could see me chewing gum to try to keep my mouth from completely drying up. I explained to anyone who would listen that it was my first time and I may just head for the door when they get started. The unsympathetic but perfectly warranted response was, "Don't faint, we won't pick you up, and if you must, don't touch anything on the way down!" And so it began, a real-life major surgery situation, patient safely asleep and the surgery starting. Suddenly, I was feeling less ill and more curious, so I got a little closer, although as I was not scrubbed there was a limit to how close I was allowed. Just as I moved a bit closer, an instrument fell from where it had been placed on top of the patient. My responses were sharp, I stuck my hand out, and caught it before it ended up on the floor. Before I had time to congratulate myself, I heard the deafening roar of the surgeon demanding the girl left the theatre... What girl...? What did she do...? Oh my Lord, he is looking directly at me. Apparently, in my bid to rescue the instrument, I breached a decontaminated area, and everyone had to pause for a short time to re-scrub, etc. I was so ashamed and, even though the theatre staff told me I wasn't the first student to do it and wouldn't be the last, I never, ever did it again. It did take me a few days to pluck up the courage to re-enter the great surgical domain known as theatre!

As the type of person who likes to chat to patients and offer reassurance, I found theatre wasn't really for me; I like my patients conscious and responsive. Although I learned the very technical aspects of theatre nursing, I was very quickly bored. Once you have seen each new operation, it becomes very routine. Then the day came when I was asked if I would like to be present at an emergency caesarean on a twin birth. Being a mum and knowing the stress of normal childbirth, I was anxious for the parents and the babies. After getting consent from the mum and dad, I scrubbed in and watched as the surgeon deftly and expertly cut through layers of fat and muscle until I could see a little arm, followed by the rest of a beautiful baby boy. After a quick cuddle with Mum, he was taken to be weighed, cleaned, etc. in the room and the second delivery continued, this time a little girl. There was no immediate cry and my colleagues worked very quietly but with a sense of urgency to help this little one. It wasn't long but seemed like a lifetime before she exercised her lungs and let Mum and Dad know she had indeed arrived. I think I probably allowed myself to breathe out at the same time. After cuddles, they both went to the special care baby unit, and I know from my subsequent enquiries they went on to gain weight and strength to happily leave for home. The miracle of birth is a delight to witness, and I am very thankful to have been allowed to be part of it. My placement continued with various speciality surgeries; eyes, orthopaedics, general surgery. As I said, although interesting, it was not for me, and I found the staff to be more technical and less people orientated. It's good that everyone has their niche; I had yet to find mine.

Medical Cardiac Ward

For my next placement I was back on the ward where I witnessed my first cardiac arrest and I was understandably a little nervous. But, with support from great staff and a great mentor, I really enjoyed this placement with no traumatic events. I witnessed the intricacies of the cardiac catheter lab watching fine wires being placed into leg arteries and guided up through to the blockages to release them. And cardioversion where someone's heart is shocked back into a normal rhythm. Again, a great mentor made me think about the role and questioned me on the four chambers of the heart and the conducting system, putting in place short learning episodes. I really felt these people wanted me to become a good nurse.

One patient on this ward made me question the idea that we do no harm. This elderly gentleman had an acute MI (myocardial infarction), more commonly known as a heart attack. He was treated outside the hospital by the paramedics and as per guidelines he was administered a thrombolytic drug to 'thin' the blood. The patient recovered from his attack but sadly a side effect of the drug was to cause a retinal bleed in the patient with some visual impairment resulting in total loss of sight. This gentleman was philosophical about the fact he was still alive but understandably frustrated by his blindness.

Although this was a cardiac ward, as with every ward, we acquired many outlying patients where there were no beds in the relevant speciality. One evening, a very confused elderly man became aggressive, agitated and violent towards the staff. This was out of character for him and derived purely from his confusion and ongoing infection. This was upsetting for the other patients and, as I came on duty the next morning, it became clear that my MI patient was very distressed. After making him a cup of tea and sitting for a chat, I realised that he had been terrified by the events of the previous evening. He could hear raised voices and anger but had no way of being able to assess the situation or whether he was in any danger due to his lack of sight. This was thought-provoking for me, as I don't think we had appreciated the impact on him. Hopefully he went on to make a different life for himself and learned to cope with his lack of sight, but if not, would he regret being given the drug that saved him?

More R & R

As a group, we enjoyed our nights out: birthdays, end of essays, 'someone broke a nail' parties. We ate many a meal whilst discussing things that would put some people off their food, but not us. One of our group, Jo, had some very coveted designer bags and always brought one out with her full of all sorts of unnecessary items, the problem was, after a wine or two (or three), the bag was abandoned, and we spent most of the night babysitting it. Eventually, she was told she was not allowed out to play unless she had a cross body bag attached to her!

We let our hair down and become irresponsible on a regular basis, enjoying the stress relief of sharing the good times and bemoaning the bad.

Short Experience Days

We were encouraged to source and request permission to work alongside various primary and secondary care disciplines to enhance our training experience and, with this in mind, I requested a few days working alongside a health visitor in the community. I worked at the GP surgery weighing babies and listening to new mums' concerns, as well as working with other health, education and voluntary agencies to support the well-being of families in the community.

However, one incident has stayed with me, which was on a visit to a family who were known to social services and the health visitors. As we approached the house, I was told a little background about alcohol and drug abuse and a family requiring immense support to look after their two little boys. As we knocked and waited for the door to be answered, we could see two little boys running around in their underwear with no sign of Mum or Dad. Eventually, Mum answered the door showing disinterest, bordering on disrespect, for the health visitor. This visit occurred because the two little boys had presented at A&E two days prior with significant burns due to being on the beach all day with no sunscreen, no protective cover and apparently no understanding of the significant resulting damage. As we left the house, I explained my feeling of horror that we were leaving the boys there as the parents had shown no remorse or indeed love for them. I was told that the family had been to court many times for neglectful behaviour, however the boys always went back as it was thought by someone that they were better off with their family. I cried that night for these two little boys and knew that I never wanted to be a social worker or health visitor if I had to accept this. Again, everyone finds their niche and I know some great social workers who strive to make a difference, and, from personal experience, as I previously noted, some who are not good at their job and perhaps needed to reflect on that and change career.

Gynaecology/Women's Health

My next placement began. My first day on this ward and I just knew that I would love it; the staff were welcoming and keen to impart their many years of experience and knowledge to me. I very quickly got involved in the pre- and post-surgery care of patients with varying conditions; breast surgery, hysterectomies, continence surgery and management of patients admitted with chronic pain from conditions such as endometriosis or chronic pelvic pain. I perfected how to catheterise and to remove a catheter with ease. I was beginning to believe that my 'want to fix things' attitude made me more of a surgical nurse than a medical nurse.

On a day looking after a four bedded bay, I had a patient who was some days past her gynae surgery and was ready for her packing to come out (medicated vaginal packing had been put in place during surgery to stop bleeding). Again, being totally inexperienced, I had no idea what this entailed and was talked through it by a staff nurse. I was told to ask the patient to take deep breaths and start to remove the packing on expiration. I tugged on a little piece of material and, all of a sudden, I felt like a magician's assistant pulling on never-ending bunting, except it wasn't out of a hat, it wasn't rainbow coloured and there was no white rabbit. My poor patient found it very uncomfortable as the packing had dried, and I was trying to gauge my speed, concentrate on her, my breathing and make her as comfortable as possible in getting the damn stuff out. I was told to think about pulling a plaster off: quick and easy. Another lesson learnt.

Another patient had a fungating breast wound, which she felt highly embarrassed about due to the smell and was understandably very emotional about her body image. These ladies with their various problems were treated on this ward with so much respect and understanding, and given the emotional support they so badly needed. There is a lot to be said for a women's health ward, although sadly due to cuts this ward has now closed and I feel fearful that future patients will not receive such dedicated care.

As I was now further into my training, a big part of this placement was learning to delegate, to have my own patients to care for and to master the art of the drug round.

Drug rounds, especially for a student, are terrifying. Even though it is supervised, you are given the responsibility of reading the drug chart and deciphering the generic names of drugs to give the right drug at the right time via the right route to the right patient, phew! On one such drug round, I gave the little pot of medication to a patient before moving on to the next, only to hear her say, "Oh, I don't usually have a yellow one." Well, Usain Bolt could not have got back to her quicker to snatch the pot out of her hand. It was not a dangerous drug she had been given, and would have caused her no harm; however, I was devastated that I had made such a mistake. There is not a nurse in this land who has not either made a mistake or had a near miss. One ward I was on introduced tabards for the nurse to wear whilst doing the drug round that said something along the lines of 'please do not disturb me or ask questions at this time, as I am concentrating on the drug round'. What a good idea.

A & E

This placement probably excited me more than any other, as well as terrifying me. There are several areas of A & E, minors, majors and resus. Self-explicable really, minors involved a lot of sprains, pains and fractures, all sorts of things in all sorts of orifices, and generally the walking wounded. Majors is again as you would expect, patients with general pain, more significant distress and concern. And then resus, a scary place for a student to be. My mentor was a very skilled nurse who had lots of education to impart, and I joined her several times in resus. I found out very quickly if I was to be of any use whatsoever, I should learn where fluids are kept, all the different syringes and needle sizes and, in general, be useful but not in the way.

An emergency call came through from the ambulance. A patient had collapsed at home, he had been resuscitated by his wife and was being brought in. The patient arrested again in the ambulance and on first arrival to resus. The team on standby are unbelievably skilled and work so well without the apparent need for direction. Of course, there is a knowledge of who is in charge and who should be doing what, but to the green student it seemed like something I would never learn. They worked tirelessly on the gentleman whilst I drew up lots of saline flushes (not to be underestimated) and for a while we got him back. At this point, a discussion was had with his wife and the consultant about the likelihood that her husband would not survive, and an explanation given of a do not resuscitate order. As I indicated previously, that means that no active CPR will be performed should he arrest, and he would be allowed to pass in a dignified and peaceful manner. As the student, I was given the task of being close to the husband and wife should she need someone and blended into the background as much as possible whilst she talked to him. She talked about his love of photography and dancing, she asked at one point if he could hear her, and I don't know for certain, but I'm told it's the last sense to go and I think talking to the unconscious patient can only help both parties. She carried on reminiscing with him until sadly his breathing laboured and stopped. Someone took her to the relatives' room to make calls and have that wonder cure, tea. In the meantime, along with a colleague, I washed the patient's face and hands before she returned. She expressed her gratitude at our efforts as it had given her a chance to say goodbye and talk to him about the good times they'd had. Over the course of my training and my professional employment, I have sometimes pondered the benefits of CPR in some cases, but I remember this patient and his wife and the benefit they had from just a little more time.

The thing about A & E is it has intense, rapid, think on your feet moments and can be emotionally as well as physically draining, but sometimes you go home feeling uplifted and just know that you made a difference.

Jean was a lady brought in from her care home. She suffered from Alzheimer's and had a fall resulting in a very deep and nasty laceration to the back of her head. Taking a confused person out of a familiar environment can cause more confusion and Jean was giving us all a lesson in the sheer volume of expletives there are; she would have blended into a rugby team dressing room without any problem. Her daughter had come with her and was very embarrassed about her mum's behaviour, which was far from her normal disposition. The doctor needed to keep Jean's head still whilst he cleaned and sutured her wound. However, she was gesticulating wildly, and it was all going horribly wrong. Her daughter, trying to calm her, reminded her of how she loved to sing, especially during the war and with the Salvation Army. Her attention duly held, I took the opportunity to gently hold her head, quietly talking to her about her favourite songs and war stories. The result was me, her daughter and Jean singing songs from before I was born (but scarily knew the words to) and so we rolled out the barrels, we visited the white cliffs of Dover and packed up our troubles at the same time as making sure Jean remained calm and steady whilst her wound was cleaned, sutured and dressed. On drawing back the curtains, we were treated to a round of applause from an audience appreciative of their temporary release of waiting room boredom (or maybe they just wanted us to stop!). Reminiscence of the past can offer some familiarity and comfort in confused patients, and I must admit I always enjoy a singsong. Some days, I just had the best job in the world.

It was not all lifesaving shifts on A & E, and some were a bit boring, nothing desperate happening, just a unit full of minor injuries, and we did have some discreet laughs, particularly with the various implements ending up in the most unusual places. One repeat admission did make me feel helpless and it was a teenage girl (boys also attended) who came into the department in DKA, diabetic ketoacidosis, which is potentially a life-threatening complication of diabetes mellitus. There can be lots of reasons for this condition, infection and poor insulin therapy being two common factors. Sadly, this young girl was identified as intentionally omitting her insulin to promote weight loss. This behaviour can be challenging, as it's often hidden and denied. Despite talks explaining the long-term damage of badly controlled diabetes and the acute DKA episodes, this girl was a regular attender in A & E. It's difficult being different when you are a teenager and want to eat/drink and be just like your friends. However, with maturity hopefully came the knowledge that, to live a happy and healthy life, acceptance of her diabetes and management of it were vital.

Of course, A & E on a Friday and Saturday night is another life. So many people who do not recognise that A & E means accident and emergency.

One particular man was brought in by paramedics having fallen in a state of inebriation and received a railing through his arm, which had to be cut through by the fire service and he came complete with metal rail in situ. The "gentleman", fair to say, was abusive, loud and generally an obnoxious drunk whose only form of communication appeared to be "geez a drink" and **** off. Now, all that we had in common was that we were both Scottish. However, this was taken by the staff to mean that I could calm him! I tried to tell him he could not have a drink and that he would have to go to theatre to have the rail removed from his arm. I offered water sponges to wet his mouth and was told again to **** off and that he wanted a real drink. Several hours passed by, the other patients having treatment were getting agitated because of him, and he showed no signs of the alcohol causing sleepiness. Eventually, I whispered in his ear in my best Scottish accent what I thought of his behaviour and that under no circumstances was he getting a drink, to which he replied, "Don't you effin' pretend to be Scottish, if ye wore, you'd know I need a drink!" I'm not sure how his behaviour changed, if at all, when he sobered up. This is the thing about A & E, very often you did not get to know what happened to the patient after they left the department. Sometimes that was frustrating and I would make a point of trying to find out on my next shift, but, in the case of my Scottish friend, sometimes it was a blessing.

In between and during placements, of course, we had study periods with our programme tutor Sarah, who was amazing at keeping us calm, getting us back on track when we were wobbling and assuring us we would pass the course. And we had clinical tutors who were maybe not quite so good. I was okay at sitting in a class and listening when I felt it was relative to my learning and that the tutor respected the fact we were all adults with many and various life experiences. But that was not always the case. Another member of my cohort Michelle and I became known as one tutor's nemesis. She shall remain nameless, but she really needed to do something other than attempt to teach. Interestingly, my essays marked by her got the fewest marks; maybe it got personal! More TMAs, more placements and generally no life, but an eye on the finish line meant I was coping.

While on placement in A & E, I spent time in the emergency admission unit, which is where, after a four hour (or so) wait, a patient was sent if they couldn't be sent to a ward. These patients could need cardiac monitoring in a bay or close attention, as conditions could deteriorate very quickly in patients not yet diagnosed.

Of course, as well as physically ill patients, we would get mentally ill patients whilst waiting for a psych review (lots of waiting for that). One regular would come in as an attempted suicide with her bags packed with make-up, candles and books. I was not sure what spa she thought was available in the afterlife she was going to! I always had a mixture of sadness for people who attempted suicide, as everyone has a story, but the revolving door patients tested me a little more. Luckily for them, and me, mental health never figured in my long-term plan; I'm all about the fixing!

Three Years In

Now into my third year of training, I was still working bank shifts to support our need to eat, working hard on my academic writing skills, as well as pretty much full-time working on placements. I never thought it would be easy, but I did feel that nursing students got a pretty bad deal compared to other uni students who are able to take part-time jobs and only attend a certain amount of time. If you take the hours worked by a student nurse on placement and the bursary they received, then it would work out about 50p an hour doing a challenging job – political views over, for now!

Two more placements left, and I was really beginning to feel like a nurse. I was learning so much and I knew, as difficult as it was, I had made the right decision in taking this steep learning curve on. Maybe I had been brave, and I was certainly a lot stronger than I thought.

Whilst on the admissions ward, a patient was admitted with shortness of breath. She was the same age as me, and her life experiences appeared to mirror some of mine; divorced, new and second relationship and lots of future plans. She had been walking with her partner and the dog and become unusually short of breath. We hit it off very well and I accompanied her to X-ray as the medical staff had suspected and wanted to confirm their thoughts that this lady had a PE (pulmonary embolism) or blood clot in her lung, which, diagnosed in time, is very treatable. Later in the shift, the consultant came to talk to her and, as a student soaking up all experiences, I went with him. What I did not expect and was not prepared for was that she had lung cancer with some spread. She was devastated, as you would expect, and I found myself desperately trying to hold back my tears and concentrate on her. She asked if I would come back in later when her partner arrived, as she wanted someone in there when she told him, before getting the consultant back to explain the plan moving forward. In the meantime, I tried to get as much information as I could to explain to them both. I felt so sad leaving the shift as all her future plans she'd shared with me would, at the very least, need to be altered. Sometimes life felt very unfair.

Sometimes, on the saddest of days, I was lucky enough to be given a little reason to smile. An elderly lady was asked by the domestic about her meal choices for that day. Her response was to ask for a little smoked salmon on brown bread with just the lightest drizzle of virgin olive oil. Not on the NHS, my lovely!

August

This is the time when new junior doctors came onto the wards and departments straight from medical school. What a huge responsibility they have to suddenly have to make the decisions as well as being incredibly tired and stressed. On more than one occasion, I came across one crying in the sluice or in an unused side room. What I would say is that the clever ones found out very quickly to get the nursing staff on side, which would make their placement so much better. More than once, a junior doctor was heard to say, "Well, I was thinking that…" and an experienced nurse finishing, "A bag of fluids, IV antibiotics and regular observations?" Never underestimate the value of the nursing staff to the medical staff, and the ones who were arrogant enough to assume superiority (and there were some), well, let's just say, sometimes help came a little slower.

Short Experience Days Again

This time I decided I would visit a volunteer-run needle exchange clinic in the community. Before visiting the exchange, I felt a little apprehensive. As much as I hate to say it, I was perhaps a little judgemental. I'd had nothing to do with addicts on a personal level and I imagined a steady stream queuing up to take advantage of the free facilities. The reality was that the programme was run from a small office and facilitated by a very friendly, knowledgeable and interesting ex-heroin addict. I learned about barrels, citric acid for mixing and various needles and sites used for injection. Everyone attending gave only their initials and date of birth, this information being used to audit service users. It was clear there were many returning and well-known characters, with some happy to stop and chat about their journey and some only interested in getting clean supplies and leaving. One particular chap was nineteen years old, and he talked with the volunteer about a methadone programme. After he left, I was told that this boy's parents had both been addicts and, as a result, his life choices had been somewhat limited.

People came and went with drug-related abscesses and stories about how nothing was their fault. I could, however, see that everyone had a story and a reason perhaps for how they succumbed to this lifestyle. My personal values remained the same after this experience but my ability to recognise that these values can often be a barrier to care was a lesson worth learning.

Hospice Care

continued working at the hospice on the bank as a healthcare assistant, firstly because I enjoyed the staff and the patients, and secondly because my bank balance diminished two weeks into a monthly paid salary. I found out there that some things just can't be explained. A lovely man had been admitted a few days earlier, as his condition was deteriorating, but he had had a good day with all of his family visiting. About thirty minutes after they all left, he asked me to call them and ask them to come back, as he just knew his time had come and he was going to die at 9pm that evening. Although I felt this was unlikely to happen in such an exact way, I telephoned his family and apologised for bothering them, but I thought they would want to know that he was agitated and told them what he was saying. They dutifully and tearfully returned and sat with him past 9pm and nothing, he remained in the same condition, enjoyed more reminiscing and sharing tales with them. Off they went home again, and he settled down to sleep after a chat and a hot drink. At 9am exactly the following morning, he passed. As I said, some things remain a mystery.

Payday Disco

Of course, it wasn't all work and no play. Every month, in the hospital social club, there were the infamous payday discos. Now, having a certain amount of maturity (well, in years, if not attitude) did not stop me joining in for a bit of a boogie. However, there was much more enjoyment to be had people watching and oh the stories I could tell, but what goes on in the disco stays in the disco! Stress relief for hardworking people.

The Big Chill

A gain, for the sake of my bank balance, I was looking for extra work, which would also give me enough time for study. A friend informed me that she went to festivals as a nurse and that there may be an opportunity for me to go. I would get paid, work twelve hours on, twelve hours off and listen to music. It was a no-brainer except I would have to sleep in a tent. I had never camped, nor had I ever wished to, but I borrowed a tent and off I went to work as a first-aider at the Big Chill festival. Forty-two thousand people camping out with supplies of permitted alcohol and unpermitted drugs, what could go wrong? Practically, we dealt with excesses of both, sprains, cuts, stings, ticks and bony injuries, some needing hospital transfer, most needing dressings and TLC. On the first day, a gentleman came to the first aid tent to have a minor cut dressed. He was a happy chap fuelled by copious amounts of alcohol and had pitched his tent and gone off drinking and socialising for that day. Unfortunately, he now couldn't remember where his tent was and, in this vast site with thousands of people, it was very unlikely he would find it. Every day he came back to have his dressing changed and to tell us he still hadn't found his tent, but every day he had made a new group of friends who allowed him to share their facilities. He was unconcerned and totally relaxed about it and we enjoyed the reciting of his stories each day. In between shifts, we had free time to watch the music. In this instance, the headliners were the Proclaimers and Lily Allen. I'm sure in the space of those few days I certainly did walk 500 miles. I came home grubby, footsore and weary, but glad of the experience. Oh, and the money! I had a vision of a lone tent standing when the site was cleared.

Next Placement: ICU

Whilst A & E excited me, ICU (intensive care unit) scared the life out of me. It is, by very definition, looking after the most vulnerable people, with life sometimes being held by a very precarious thread. It is a scary place, full of wires, monitors and strange noises. On the upside, there is almost one-to-one nursing a lot of the time, but that is because these patients really need it, and I was worried I wouldn't be up to that; would I trip, as I am and always have been incredibly clumsy, and detach someone from some life-saving equipment or pull a tube out or give medicine into the wrong port, as there were so many? Eventually, I became a little more settled with help again from a great team of people.

There are always patients from every speciality who strike a chord and here we had a patient who was a policeman who had developed Guillain-Barré syndrome. This is a rare but serious condition affecting the nerves. It is treatable, and most people will eventually make a complete recovery, but it can be life-threatening and some can be left with long-term problems. This patient was paralysed from the neck down and had very limited ability to communicate. This was a fit young family man who, through a viral infection, became life threatened. Following a long time of mechanical breathing and tracheostomies, I witnessed the final stages of his recovery during my placement, and he was eventually sent to a rehab place with the intention that he would recover fully in time. His wife and family were unfailing in visiting and attention, despite him at times being less than grateful, due to his frustrations, I'm sure.

Everyone on ICU who is unconscious had a diary by their bed for staff and relatives to write in each day to remind them when it was all over about what had been happening to them. Many patients wake with no recollections and can blank out months, others wake with stories of nightmares and stressful situations. It reassures that you should always explain to patients what you are doing and why, and never, ever assume they can't hear you or aren't frightened by the lack of knowing what is happening to them. During my time there, I witnessed families being given life-changing news about their loved ones and the raw grief of loved ones when the expected and unexpected death happens. Once again, I don't believe this will be my area of choice to work in.

Academia

I have never been great at exams. I get a tickly cough and a dry mouth, suddenly having the inability to remember my name. The years have not changed this, and so I was apprehensive to say the least about my forthcoming BIG exam. I had to pass, as this, alongside my coursework, would determine whether I qualified as a registered nurse.

I like people, I like to know what is happening to them with disease progression and trauma, however I am at a loss with the intricacies of synapses and atoms. To prepare for this major exam, I did what all sensible people do. I went to Alicante with Tracy (who had become a great friend). We discussed taking notepads, books and reference points with us and would test each other on the points we thought would come up in the exam. In practice, we sunbathed, drank wine and basically enjoyed life. On our last day, we discussed that the party was over, and we needed to do some serious revising. At the airport, we were told the flight was cancelled due to fog. We had no money left, but luckily could get a lift back to Tracy's villa for the night. Travelling back, we decided that, as we had spent up, we would spend that evening revising and talking about our imminent exam. Fortunately, or unfortunately, we met some friends again who offered to subsidise a last night in La Luz (a bar, a pole and music, what could go wrong?) and our resolve quickly diminished. Returning from Spain, it suddenly seemed that it wasn't a good idea at all. I had learned *dos vino tinto por favor*, but very little about human biology. I spent the next week resolutely pasting Post-it notes all over my kitchen cupboards with buzz words on them. I wrote and rewrote scenarios until I could get it down to a few words. I was a stressed-out mother in her fifties by that time with a menopausal brain, thinking what on earth possessed me to think I could do this. I had nights where I cried myself to sleep thinking I had just been deluded to think I could do this course and become the registered nurse I wanted to be.

The Day of the Exam

We travelled to the venue en masse and met for coffee beforehand. No one could eat, there were Rescue Remedy pastilles being shared and I had my vial of it that was popped on my tongue every two seconds (can you overdose on it?).

Multiple choice questions gave way to the all-important essay question. There are many things about that exam that I have forgotten, except this question:

"For breakfast, Mr Smith had toast, cheese and tomato – explain the process from the mouth through the digestive tract of each component."

Now, the digestive tract is from the mouth to the large intestine, that's a long way to remember. What happens to the carbs and the protein? Is it the hydrochloric acid or the pepsin, or both that are needed? … Couldn't he just have had porridge?

After three hours, we came out of the exam in stunned silence, everyone agreeing not to talk about it for fear of knowing we had messed up. The tapas bar called, where we had carbs, protein and wine. A waiting game began.

Looking to the Future

I n the meantime, it was time to apply for jobs (in the hope that I had passed the exam), and my first choice was the gynae ward where I had been on my placement. I knew that if I worked on that ward I would have so much support from the staff and it would be a great grounding in drug rounds, surgical procedures and would enhance my knowledge in this field. I applied for a newly qualified position and got an interview; I was so excited. A few days before my interview, I started to feel unwell and assumed it was probably nerves and exhaustion; however, I ended up taking up a bedspace in EAU (emergency assessment unit) with swine flu! As soon as I started to feel just a little better, I telephoned the ward to explain and asked if there was any possibility of changing my interview date or having a telephone interview. Okay, I was contagious, but they knew me. Unfortunately for me, the dates are set in stone and do not allow individual circumstance to dictate. I was upset and felt I had failed at the first hurdle, as well as feeling unwell.

Picking myself up, I applied for a job on EAU. I knew the manager wasn't keen on newly qualified, but I went into pester mode and eventually got an interview and my first job as a registered nurse.

A Real Nurse

To graduate as a registered nurse is right up there with some of the most important moments in my life. I still had imposter syndrome and a fear of failure, but on the day of my graduation, I felt invincible. I couldn't believe that I was going to walk across that stage, albeit precariously, with my cap and gown and celebrate becoming a registered nurse. Both my daughters were in the audience, as was my partner (the one I felt may be special way back at the beginning of this journey) and they all supported me wholeheartedly in this amazing achievement. As they called my name, I could hear my daughter call out, "Go Mum!" and I had a tear in my eye. What a day! I came back to the Bay for a surprise meet up, arranged by my man with my longest and best friend, with cake and champagne. Oh, my goodness, I had done it.

Cast your mind back to my first day on the 'bank' and the tetraplegic man. Here I was, about to start my first day as a registered nurse in that very department, oh how long ago that seemed!

Another brand-new uniform, but this time I was a qualified nurse with all the responsibility that goes with that. I was remembered by staff from my placement there and had a mentor to guide me as I continued this learning curve, but I felt amazing. I am home, this is who I am, Staff Nurse McGregor.

First Position: EAU (Emergency Admissions Unit) Linked to A & E

The department had single rooms, bays of four and a high dependency bay, which was used for the most poorly patients, including those who required cardiac monitoring.

Accident and emergency is not to be confused with anything and everything, which I soon realised was a fact that not all of the general public were familiar with. More of that later.

The transition from student nurse to qualified nurse was a shock to the system. As a student, I felt it acceptable to ask for advice when I was unsure and, although I had an incredible support network in the more qualified nurses and unit managers, I felt the weight of responsibility bearing down on me. As I've mentioned before, I would never underestimate that the patient assumes that you know what is best for him/her and will, in the most part, trust implicitly in what you say.

Night Shifts

Night shift is a strange time in a hospital environment. It is less busy, fewer investigations are being conducted and, once everyone is settled for the night, it can have an eerie feeling about it. In fact, there was a book going round the hospital asking people to document any strange occurrences or ghost stories they may have had. It may surprise you how many there were.

One night shift, at about 2am, two teenagers were brought in to A & E with unexplained chest pain. After ECGs and bloods did not show anything untoward, they were transferred to our department for an overnight stay and to be on cardiac monitoring, just to be sure nothing was being missed. These two boys had clearly been partying and drinking prior to admission and were disruptive and noisy until they eventually fell asleep. With regular observations through the night, and at one point a shoe full of vomit (I did not dodge it quickly enough), there was no further indication of chest pain. Unremarkably, in the morning, they ate a hearty breakfast and wondered if I could get the ambulance to take them home. My assumption was they had spent up, had no taxi fare home, called an ambulance with 'chest pain' and managed to get a bed for the night. Did I get them transport home? What do you think? I wonder if they ever considered the cost of their stay or the impact on a potentially vulnerable person having to wait for a bed?

By far the majority of people who present at hospital are scared, concerned and just need reassurance and treatment. But there are the drunks and others who abuse your good intentions, allowing – actually, expecting – to be cleaned up and given a bed for the night, only to vomit and sh*t on themselves with the expectation that someone will do it all again, uncomplaining. Like I said before, we are not angels, just people trying to do the best job they can and sometimes getting frustrated with the expectations on the NHS.

Every shift I came into the department in my new uniform was daunting initially. I worried about what I would be faced with, would I make the right decisions for my patients, would I get through it without killing anyone? As you walk through A & E and into EAU, it has a special feel, different from wards. It has an atmosphere of tension, business, a plethora of vulnerable people all looking for someone to reassure and treat where appropriate. I think what I most loved about it and what most excited me about working there (and probably most scared me) was that you never knew what you would be facing each shift. Mostly patients would arrive from A & E after their four-hour (ish) wait and have a bed whilst continuing to be investigated or until they went to the appropriate ward (providing there were beds). I routinely cannulated, took blood and catheterised like a real nurse. Catheterisation was always a bit of a challenge, a skill that I really wanted to be expert at, but sometimes it just didn't go to plan. Males were easier: one entry point. Some anatomy in females, especially in the older patients, is a bit lax and there is more than one orifice there, so occasionally it would not work to plan and the whole aseptic kit needed to be discarded and attempted again.

Orifices

have witnessed some very strange objects in some very strange places, with a fair amount of people 'falling' off a stool whilst putting shopping away or cleaning out cupboards onto an upturned object (very regularly a deodorant can), which ended up in their rectum. Now quite why these people were putting their shopping away naked was beyond me. One patient attended with a vibrator stuck inside his rectum. His X-rays showed clearly the batteries were still going and many a joke was made about the Duracell bunny (not in front of the patient, I have to say). Laughing at patients was maybe not the right thing to do, but the dark humour of medical staff is one I hold dear. There is a cautionary tale regarding this patient, though, as he almost perforated his bowel and needed surgery. When he came round from the anaesthetic, he asked for the vibrator back, as he would have to put it back before his girlfriend got back from a weekend away as she didn't know he used it. UUUUGGGGHHHH! I hope he used more than a wet wipe.

Another random patient who springs to mind is the one who decided to superglue his foreskin just to see what happened! Mmmm, you won't be able to pee, and it will really hurt. As my mother used to say, "There's nowt so queer as folk!"

As I got more confident in my ability to nurse without accidentally killing someone, I relaxed a little bit more into the role. Handover, as I learned in my training, needed to be concise. By the end of your shift, everyone was tired and anxious to handover and go home. One nurse on handover would routinely tell everyone how many people had called for a certain patient or what they ate for dinner or what colour nightie they were wearing. Not sure anyone ever explained to her the definition of concise, and I used to dread having to take handover from her. Many a time after a twelve-hour shift, I would go home and think about whether I told them about someone needing fluids or meds or messages from home. I usually had but sometimes I would call the ward just to check. We are not infallible and there is a lot going on. It's a hard job with the constant juggling of tasks and trying to keep all the balls in the air whilst looking as though you are calm and completely in control.

Crash Calls

ooking back to my first hospital arrest where I cut tubes and looked on helplessly, I have since attended quite a few. Not as many in hospital as you think; as I have said, everyone is so closely monitored, we hopefully catch a problem before it happens. The adrenaline when that alarm goes, the only time you should see a nurse running, is like nothing else and your brain just goes into automatic pilot at the time, getting oxygen on, doing chest compressions, etc. It's only afterwards that you start to think about that person and what they have just gone through, sometimes successfully, sometimes sadly not.

I don't think I ever got complacent, but I think that was a good thing. It wasn't all work. We had leaving dos, starting dos, weddings, birthdays, 'any excuse' dos, and I worked with an amazing team of people from wonderful senior nurses such as Nicky, an inspirational leader who was knowledgeable and never failed to pass that knowledge on or to help when she could, before a junior nurse asked, where it was required, to HCAs who could still run rings round this newly qualified nurse but who were so supportive and helpful to me. Thank you, Nina and Lou, who had my back. I loved working in this fast-paced environment and being the age I was didn't seem to deter me, but many a time I came home after a twelve-hour shift pretty much on my knees, wondering why I had left it so late in life to do it. I do strongly believe that past life experiences help develop skills, so no regrets, it was the right time and the right place to be.

Moving Time

By this time, my girls were either at uni, had left home or were travelling and I was mostly on my own. My special person, Bob, was still on the scene and lived in Bristol. We made time at weekends and on leave to see each other, which was a lovely distraction, but sometimes when I had a particularly difficult shift or dealt with someone else's emotional stress, it was quite nice to come home to self-thinking time and recharge the batteries.

In time, we had a decision to make about me moving to Bristol where his family and work were more accessible, or staying in the Bay and at the hospital that had been such an important part of my journey. I discussed this at length with my girls and my friends and decided to take the plunge and move at some point in the not-too-distant future. After much travelling to view houses and plan our future life, we bought a house and put the wheels in motion to move. I made the difficult decision to leave the department I loved, the hospital I loved and the area I loved to move to Bristol to enable us to be together properly.

I had looked, whilst I was still in Torbay, for an appropriate role in Bristol, but there was nothing similar to what I had been doing. Or maybe I was just scared about going into a big hospital without the familiarity and support I'd had. A role was advertised in a brand-new treatment centre very close to where we had bought our bungalow. It was a privately owned company but treating NHS patients. I applied and was offered the role as an outpatient nurse with eight-till-five hours, enabling me to set up our home, make friends and spend time with our newly acquired cockapoo puppy.

New Challenges

A private treatment centre was very, very different from the NHS, and also very different from a private hospital. Firstly, at interview, I had to negotiate my salary… I had always been on a particular band in the NHS and there were points to get to the top of your band and promotions to move to the next. At interview, I said what salary I thought would be fair and got it. It turns out I'm pretty sh*t at negotiating. We all earned different amounts, regardless of work ethics or capabilities; a lesson learned.

There was a lead nurse, who was given the role because another department wanted to let him go, and a team of agency nurses earning a fortune for very little work, but I would take my badly negotiated salary, do my job and go home every evening. It was okay, but I never really had that 'real nurse' feeling dealing with outpatient appointments.

I have always been about trying to offer the best service you can, whatever job you do, so when I started to see areas that could be improved, I did what

I always do and jumped in feet-first to try to enhance the service. It was a very dictatorial management style at the centre. I was used to NHS management where, if a problem was identified, it would be discussed, and the appropriate people would each put views forward about how best to manage it (most of the time). At the treatment centre, if an issue was escalated, it was usually met with 'don't bring me problems, bring me solutions'. Sometimes management needed to contribute to the solutions, but I'll leave that there.

Clinics consisted of orthopaedic, ENT, gynae, surgical and urology. Most of the consultants were from an Eastern European background, most were very nice, but one in particular would drive in at Dick Dastardly speed forty-five minutes late for clinic every day, leaving poor patients with almost an hour extra to wait before it even got started, but no one seemed to think this was a problem except me. I spoke to him and explained how the patients must feel and maybe if he had trouble getting there for 8:30, we could rearrange the clinic to start later. He looked at me with a cross between contempt and horror at my daring to question him and never actually spoke to me again; arrogance at its very best. Even after complaining to management, he was never requested to get to work on time.

Of the clinics we had, the consultants, especially surgical and ENT, would require examination tools, gloves, gel, etc., and had to keep asking the staff to get things. While I was there and now outpatient lead (a better salary negotiated), I allocated one HCA per room and had a trolley laid out with all necessary equipment as standard. The appreciation from these consultants was worth all the negativity from some staff and I had many emails in thanks from them.

Not all staff were on board with this, and one particular HCA was obstructive, to say the least. At one point, after being asked to set up the trolley, I went to the room, and it wasn't set up. When I called him into the office to question him, I was told, "Someone must have it in for me and dismantled it after I'd done all the work." As this person talked the talk, he was allowed to get away with so much more from the powers that be. Some people brighten up a room just by leaving it.

I loved the urodynamics clinic and even went to Newcastle to learn the art of urodynamic testing. This process looks at how well the lower urinary tract, the bladder, sphincters and urethra work to store and release urine. With this explanation in mind, you will appreciate that my patients consisted mostly of ladies who were experiencing some degree of urinary incontinence. This may be due to an overactive bladder, stress incontinence or urge incontinence.

The process involves inserting probes linked to equipment to trace the filling and voiding of the bladder. Once the probes are in place, the patient may be asked to cough, laugh, star jump and run on the spot, so not dreadfully dignified, but to these patients I'm sure worth it if the source of their incontinence could be identified and managed. My biggest problem whilst conducting these tests was they made me want to pee!

Disillusioned

As time passed, I was getting more disillusioned with the service that appeared to be very money orientated and would do pretty much anything to reach targets to maintain the NHS funding. In time, an OPD (outpatient manager) was appointed (another transfer from an internal department!). On paper, she appeared to have all the necessary attributes and I vowed to support her in any way I could, UNTIL she tried to ECG a patient by placing the pads on the right side of a patient's chest. Now, even the dullest tool in the box knows the heart is on the left side, and this was a very senior (in theory) nurse. After several more issues, I raised concerns about safety to the head of nursing, who asked me just to 'be her friend' and guide her. Here we had an equivalent Band 7 nurse on approximately 20k more than me. Several more incidents on, I again approached the head of nursing, as I felt an accident was waiting to happen. Long story short, for the first time in my life, after almost two years there, I resigned without a job to go to.

Approximately seven months later, an avoidable incident did happen, and she was sacked.

It wasn't all bad. They did focus on trying to be seen to be the best, so I had courses on physical assessment skills, route cause analysis looking into 'never events' (as it says on the tin, these were adverse events that should never have happened, but do because human error can happen in any walk of life) and general management courses (although these appeared to be the ability to devise meetings to discuss previous meetings and adjourn events for future meetings).

Back to a Hospital Environment

Onwards and upwards, there was a temporary six-month role going at the city hospital for a VTE nurse. I had to google it before I applied. Venous thromboembolism is a term referring to blood clots in the veins. It is an underdiagnosed and serious – yet preventable – medical condition that can cause death and disability. The role basically involved trying to negate or minimise inpatient thrombosis, usually caused by a patient not being mobilised quickly enough or prescription blood thinners being missed. There had been a big drive into this, and new forms printed on which admitting doctors must assess each patient and prescribe medication where appropriate.

The role, if I chose to take it, was to go round the wards checking these forms, checking the dose had been given, making sure compression stockings or aids to keep the blood circulating were being used and to encourage patients to mobilise where possible. Speaking to the admitting doctors where information was missing was also an important part of the role and most (ish) were accepting of the advice, but I did meet, on a regular basis, arrogance and contempt again. Now, coming from Glasgow and a family of four older brothers, I grew up with a pretty thick skin and an ability to speak up for myself, so I was okay with this and took the role.

It got me used to working in a new hospital environment and the six months went past without too much abuse from doctors. I also in this time took on a teaching role devising a dreaded PowerPoint presentation and delivering it to new staff before they got let loose on the wards. I enjoyed teaching and decided I would attend night school and take a PPTLS (preparing to teach in the lifelong sector) course, hoping that one day it would be helpful in other roles. So, now it was time to look for a new role whilst taking on extra training to teach.

Oh and by the way, I had always thought if I was a nurse I would want to volunteer in a less fortunate country, to challenge myself, my skills and my compassion by nursing somewhere without the comforts and accessibility of the equipment I'd had. So here I go again, with the blessing of my other half and my children, I researched available options and applied to go to Cambodia on a three-week healthcare outreach programme taking place the following year. It involved self-funded travel to Cambodia to work on a volunteer basis to be part of an ongoing programme to teach aspects of healthcare and to generally do whatever was needed.

The PTLLS course was a ten-week evening class course. In my group were eleven other people, all from different backgrounds, who wanted to be able to teach their craft, such as origami, craft beer production, wood carving, foreign languages, to name just a few. We learned the different learning styles, visual, auditory and kinaesthetic, sometimes a mix of all. I found it interesting to know why a PowerPoint may be crucial for some and absolute hell for others and again confirmed my learning style as activist, although as a nurse maybe it should have been reflective? At the end of the course, a teaching plan had to be written and delivered to the others in the class. For some reason, everyone thought they would like to know how to give an injection. They weren't medical and, as far as I knew, they weren't drug addicts, so why? But I duly obliged, and my session was on anaphylaxis and how to inject adrenaline if called upon to do it. The person in the class who was most desperate for me to do this promptly fainted at the first sign of the needle being unsheathed... go figure.

Thinking about transferrable skills, and probably having seen too many episodes of *Doctors*, I decided a GP practice nurse was going to be my niche. No previous knowledge of smears, immunisations, chronic disease management, but every day is a school day, right?

The Nurse Will See You Now

applied to a local village GP practice and miraculously they took me on. I was going to love getting to know people and seeing them on a regular basis, being a big part of the community and working pretty much autonomously in my clinic room; what could go wrong? I told them at interview about my volunteering plans and they were happy for me to have the required time off; win, win.

So, back to courses, with cervical sampling being a biggy. I had to learn the theory and, as you can't really practise on each other (that would be weird), it was a 'see one, do one, teach one' moment. I loved the challenge of getting the correct cells from the correct area whilst being as gentle as possible with the speculum and trying to put people at ease. I had to have a large number of correct sampling results before I could be passed as competent. I can assure you, ladies, we are all the same, there is no need to be embarrassed and IT SAVES LIVES. Next, child immunisation. This is led by public health and, after doing the required immunisation course, I was let loose on the baby and child population of our practice area. Thursday was imms (immunisation) day and the constant pressure to check, re-check and triple-check the paperwork to ensure the correct medication at the correct dose was given to the correct age-appropriate child was horrendous. Some practices had two nurses doing it, ours had me! I wholeheartedly believe in our immunisation programme, but I found it hard to deal with the parents in tears as I subjected their child to pain, even if it was a best interest issue. One gentleman, who I assumed to be quite intelligent, informed me that he wouldn't have his twin babies vaccinated as, "No one gets polio these days." As I said, 'assumed' intelligence. I still dislike Thursdays.

A teenage girl came for her HPV vaccine (human papillomavirus) only to panic at the last minute and pull her arm away, resulting in a needlestick injury to me! It is such an important vaccine protecting against cervical cancer and some head and neck cancers that I was keen to support her to have the vaccine, so I asked her to return with someone to support her and put some headphones in with relaxing music and we would get it done. The following week, she returned, Dad in tow. I asked her to lay on the couch and pop her music in whilst dad sat at the desk. She was still very nervous and difficult to inject, but she managed it. As I turned around, however, Dad was on the floor.

A lot of the practice nurse's job is chronic disease

management, leg ulcers, smoking cessation and weight control. One patient that springs to mind was morbidly obese and had weeping leg ulcers. She attended the surgery every week to have both legs in four-layer bandaging. The rationale for this was that the compression reduced the healing time of leg ulcers. The layers usually comprised of orthopaedic wool, crepe bandage, elastic bandage and a final layer of cohesive dressing. As you can imagine, this is massively time-consuming to do, first bathing the leg and then applying the bandaging. This lady had been told that her weight was having a massive impact on her general health and mobility, but to be honest she enjoyed coming in; it was like a social event, telling me about all her neighbours' gossip, whom I neither knew nor cared about, and the sugar craft classes she went to twice a week and ate the products of her efforts. She would tell me she didn't know why she was so heavy as she ate like a sparrow. I didn't feel able to say that a sparrow is known to eat twice its body weight in food. What an expensive, avoidable state and mindset she had got herself into.

Smoking cessation was challenging, not least when I had a patient in clinic who let me go through the whole spiel about choices in patches, gum, sprays, etc., to assist in smoking cessation, before telling me he didn't smoke! "So why are you here?"

"Well, I started vaping and now it's costing me too much, so I need help."

Of course, there were the regulars coming in for their blood tests and I did indeed get to know them. One gentleman who was on a blood thinning drug came routinely for blood tests to check his levels were correct. He was a lovely man, living with his brother. Neither had ever married and they looked after each other. Coming for his blood test one day, he fell in the car park. The first I knew of this was when I went to the desk and saw him sitting there with his brother, paper tissues held to his profusely bleeding face (the blood thinners obviously do what you expect them to do and thin the blood, therefore making bleeding a risk). The GP breezed by and said I had better take him to my room to deal with him. I have to say at this point he was a typical old-fashioned GP who owned the practice as his father had before him and did not like change or inconvenience. One HCA who worked there had also been there forever and basically did exactly as she wanted to the point of being obstructive when she felt like it. Halfway along the corridor, I took a look at my patient's face and asked the HCA to get the GP as this patient was peri-arrest (about to have a cardiac arrest). She decided that it was the right time to ask me why I thought that, as said GP was busy and couldn't I deal with it?! I reiterated my request, got the patient on the couch, called an ambulance and, following the predicted arrest, started CPR. I was joined by two of the GPs, but alas we could not get him back, despite us and then the paramedics trying. His poor brother, still sitting in the waiting room unaware, had to be told by me that his brother had gone. Now, all the courses in the world about breaking bad news do not tell you how not to cry too. This poor man had a lifestyle just around him and his brother, his distress was palpable, and my fingernails dug into clenched hands helped to stem my tears. The HCA made the paramedics and the GP a cup of tea, I was left to clean the bloodbath of a room without tea and, no time for reflection or debrief, my clinic continued.

I didn't think practice nurse was my niche. Would I ever find it? I enjoyed the active smear taking, bloods and minor injuries, but struggled with a lack of willingness to go with the times (pretty floral curtains around cubicles run up by a GP on her sewing machine at home instead of disposable curtains for infection control) and a belief that if things weren't broken don't fix them, and don't rock the boat even if there was a better and safer way of doing things.

Ten months into this post, it was time for me to take leave for my volunteering project. I was intent on going alone when I booked it. Sometimes I wondered if I was brave, as I kept being told, or naïve, or reckless. Whatever it was, I just knew I wanted to take every opportunity open to me as a nurse. That's the thing about nursing, you can go off in so many directions. It took so much to get there, I wanted to live my dream without any regrets.

The idea was that you made your own way to

Cambodia and let the organisers know when you would arrive, meet a cohort of nurses over there and become a team. But, a few months after I booked it, my very good friend Jacqui decided she would come too. She was also a nurse and was looking for a challenge after having a particularly difficult few years personally. I was so pleased that I would have company on the long journey over and be able to share my experiences with Jacqui.

Cambodia

Volunteering is not cheap! Firstly, we had to have a list of vaccinations; yellow fever (don't think I will ever use the phrase 'it's just a little scratch' again), dengue fever, typhoid, hep B, hep A and rabies (although we decided against that one); expensive and painful. Also, we had to arrange anti-malarial medication and book our flights. Fortunately, we had very good friends, who, together with Bob, arranged a race night to raise funds for us, and my amazing niece Maureen arranged an eighties night back in Glasgow, which was massively successful and full of generous people. Again, I felt a bit of a fraud. People kept saying it was special and brave. It didn't feel brave, I just felt excited, and the money raised, together with our own personal savings, meant we were almost there.

Prior to going, research and programme information showed poor eyesight was a problem, as well as teaching children the importance of dental hygiene, handwashing and caring for themselves in any way they could. Armed with this knowledge, we bought a ridiculous number of reading glasses from the pound shop, the same ridiculous number of toothbrushes, and a pleading letter to Colgate resulted in a huge box of sample tubes arriving at my home free of charge.

Eventually packed, we had medication for constipation, diarrhoea, antihistamines, sunscreen, cagoules, DEET for clothes and DEET for skin (I was not entirely happy about putting something on my skin that could melt plastic, but equally I did not want to get ill, so no plastic wearing). Jacqui had a model penis, condoms, latex gloves and lubricant (sexual health promotion and not desperation). Everything packed, unpacked and repacked into my backpack, I struggled to get it all in, which was a little bit annoying, as most of it wouldn't be coming back with me.

I was a little apprehensive about the inability to contact home, as it would be rather sporadic due to signal issues in camp, but the support of my family meant everything to this dream of mine.

The first part of the journey was a thirteen-hour flight, then a stop off for seven hours in Kuala Lumpur and a remaining five-hour flight. I tried to concentrate on a book I was reading about the Khumer Rouge and then a film about an autistic child. Jacqui, meanwhile, was happily watching *Despicable Me*!

On arrival, we had a two-night stop in Siem Reap, but to be honest, I just wanted to get to camp. I would never underestimate the luxury of hot water and flushing toilets again. In the areas we had seen since arrival, 40% of people were below the WHO poverty indicator, but in the village camps we were going to, it would be around 85%. 70-75% of inhabitants around during the troubles suffered with PTSD, leading to a high incidence of alcoholism and domestic abuse. Unsurprisingly (after several near misses), road accidents are the highest cause of death, followed by HIV/AIDS, then landmines. What the hell was I doing here? I was brave, I was strong, I may have been deluded.

Camp was, as we expected, basic. There was no indication that if we said, "I'm not a celebrity get me out of here," that anything would happen. Each outdoor (yes outdoor) 'room' has a very thin mattress and a mosquito net. We did have a roof, so some shelter, at least. There were two compost toilets in camp, into which you threw down a bucket of sawdust after doing your necessary task. To be honest, this was actually more tolerable than the chemical toilets at the festival I had worked at. The food was basically rice and noodles at every meal, which was cooked for us by Sunny, a local young boy, and NO wine! Sunny was employed by the NGO and charity, but we were mostly healthcare professionals there to make a difference, promoting health and well-being, so no complaints, right? The best part of something like this was to live like a local and appreciate their struggles.

The first night in camp, it was raining all night.

What was that all about? I had sunscreen, I thought I would go home tanned, svelte and rejuvenated. It was cold, a rooster had been 'singin' since 4am and at six it was time to get up for a shower, aka a plastic bag of ice-cold water hung on a hook and attached to a shower head.

Meeting the Locals

The first village trip was to a school where there were about fifty children, some in a school uniform, some in rags. We had fun teaching them how to wash hands after touching animals. We laughed and joked with them, giving them toothbrushes and toothpaste. Almost every child had bleeding gums. They just loved to get the simplest of gifts and were so appreciative. Head lice and worms were a problem with these kids, but apart from using a cattle prod (Jacqui's idea), we had to just hope the little buggers wouldn't transfer to us.

We visited mums and babies in villages where, after using their one tin of supplied milk powder, if they had no breast milk, normally due to malnutrition, mothers were trying to give newborn babies starch water from the rice in the hope it would offer some nutrition. It didn't, and many a mum lost her baby. What I wanted to do was go and buy lots of milk, but it was not allowed to happen. There appeared to be lots of dogs around, not exactly treated as pets, but not totally feral either. I had wished at this point we hadn't decided against the rabies jab and tried as much as possible to stay away from them. One pregnant young girl was due her baby imminently and, when asked what would happen when she went into labour (these villages were a long way from civilisation), she said she would get on the back of her friend's motorbike, and they would drive three hours to the nearest hospital... in labour! Oh my goodness, can you imagine doing that?

We visited and worked at diabetic clinics giving out many pairs of free glasses. The look on someone's face when they could suddenly see to read was amazing. Funnily enough, it was the men who loved the flowery Dame Edna Everage styles. My ability to manually take blood pressures came in handy, with no tech there. We dispensed diabetic medication subsidised by charities in local community clinics attended by many people who had walked a long way to be seen.

When not taking part in some health promotion, we did a bit of bricklaying for a new teachers' block at our nearest school. This was a school of 700 pupils with two toilets (squatting holes in the ground, as had most of the areas we went to); beyond my comprehension. About 100 yards down a dirt path and across the road was a toilet block built for some dignitary or other who would be or had been passing by at some point, there were approximately eight toilets in the male and the female areas, all spotlessly clean, with flushing water and handwashing facilities. The children nor the teachers were allowed to use them! We witnessed little children, four and six, fishing with their hands in murky waters for anything edible and playing with a machete on a stick (like a hobby horse) waiting for Mum to come back (a four-mile walk) from the paddy fields where she was trying to earn a living for her children.

I am going to condense this journey, as not just one person sticks in my mind, but all of them. The acceptance of having so little, the fear and apprehension about trying to get anything better due to the war when supposed intelligent people (those who wore glasses and those who could write were just a couple of examples) were executed. I still find it amazing that this happened in the seventies. I was a teenager, why didn't I know anything about it? We went to the floating villages where kids basically got into round tin baths to fish. I wondered how they managed when the water level dropped as it did and the riverbed was dry. Such beautiful, hard-working and accepting people.

The weekend before we came home, we visited the infamous killing fields and the memorial in place was peaceful and serene, but the vision of the killing tree where babies were sent to death by beating against it was incomprehensible. Loudspeakers were high on the trees and were used to play music during the killing years to drown out the screams of the suffering. In just three years, eight months and twenty days, the Pol Pot regime managed to kill nearly three million people. S-21 prison housed the memories, and, thanks to some historians, the photos of the people kept and tortured just waiting for their execution at the killing fields. The feeling of oppression was heavy and almost tangible. It's no surprise there was distrust and reticence amongst some of the people to try and improve their lot.

On free time, we visited the many temples and saw wonderful displays of opulence at the royal palace. It just didn't sit comfortably with me when we had just witnessed such extreme poverty. Phnom Penn was bustling, with the extremes of wealth and poverty never more obvious.

I enjoyed my challenge. I wish we could have done more nursing, but the government was very reluctant to accept anything for their people. We did the little bit we could, and I accepted I couldn't change the world, but it didn't stop me wanting to.

When the time came to return home, I knew that a GP practice nurse was not for me. The adventure to Cambodia brought home to me even more how fortunate we were to have the NHS and how much we need to promote individual responsibility where appropriate. I wondered if I would ever find my niche. Maybe it had been in the emergency admissions unit, which seemed like a lifetime ago. I went back to the surgery but six months later, when a role came up in the hospital for a bowel cancer screening specialist, I knew it was for me. My niche was definitely somewhere in a hospital setting and I was passionate about promoting the health of the nation. The responsibility for our healthy futures could not just lie with the NHS. I researched the BCSP (bowel cancer screening programme) and applied for the role. The requirements were some experience of endoscopy procedure – tick – ability for autonomous working – tick – and a knowledge of the programme. I read and researched it all. The interview went well, and I was offered the role. Three months of notice (yes, three) later, I was able to leave the surgery and move on.

My Niche

I was again working in a large teaching hospital but since I had temporarily done the VTE (venous thromboembolism) project post, the building and layout was more familiar to me. The post of SSP (specialist screening practitioner) involved going to Liverpool University within the year and taking a study module in bowel cancer screening, learning in great depth about polyps, cancers, other bowel diseases/disorders, writing essays on comorbidities (health conditions that people live with which may have an impact on screening) and learning in the role.

All this training would be done over approximately eight months, two full weeks in Liverpool and the rest self-led study, the submission of a portfolio and a final exam. All whilst working full time and learning my role on the shop floor, so to say. I'm not sure why I felt the need to do this to myself, but there was a part of me, as I said previously, that just wanted to grab every opportunity, and maybe a part of it was trying to prove that I actually was good enough.

It was a small team I worked with, and the role had essentially three parts. The general public were sent a screening kit from the age of sixty to seventy-four, which involved collecting a small sample of stool and sending it back to a central hub, where it would be analysed for microscopic blood. A positive test resulted in a referral to the bowel screening team responsible for the area they lived in. An appointment would be made for them to attend a positive assessment clinic with an SSP (me), where we would go into great detail around their general health and well-being, medication, etc., before telling them all about what a screening colonoscopy entailed, which was basically some preparation (pretty awful tasting) to empty their bowel and then a colonoscope into the rectum to look all the way around the bowel looking for any obvious cause of the blood, polyps or abnormalities. The test can be uncomfortable, and sedation is offered. We are so lucky in the UK to have screening programmes available on the NHS, cervical, breast, prostate, AAA and bowel; of all the programmes, I believe bowel screening to be absolutely live saving. I'm passionate about the service that is offered and will always be an advocate for it. So, three parts: assessment clinic, attending colonoscopy procedures to support and advocate for the patient and obtaining results for any polyps or tissue removed and initiating results clinics and follow-up plans. One in ten people with a positive test may have a bowel cancer, but the majority will either have polyps, which can be removed, or no indication about why their test was positive. So, again, there was an element of breaking bad news, but mostly just having people who were so appreciative of such a good service and peace of mind. Maybe I had found niche number two. Being a programme invited by age, there were a great variety of people and I have always been a people person, so what was not to love? The endoscopists I worked with were excellent; well, one may have been a little pedantic, however a great 'scopist nonetheless. The programme initially involved fifty-five-year-olds for a part examination (called a bowel scope). Decided not on a positive test but just age related, this involved having an enema – a process that involves the patient inserting a plastic tube into the rectum and squeezing the contents of an attached bottle of fluid to clear the lower part of the bowel. However, this was abandoned during the pandemic (more on this later) and was never reinstated, the plan being to bring the age down to fifty eventually, so that everyone over that age would get a full examination.

Patients (although I shouldn't really call them that as they are not unwell) never fail to surprise me.

Mr P, young and fit, had received an invitation to have a bowel scope and sent the preparation, which would produce a bowel movement, to administer at home. On admission, he said how awful it had tasted and I had to really think, as I'd thought he was on a bowel scope list, not a full colonoscopy. But, yes, he had drunk the enema through the 'straw' (the insertion tube to go into the rectum). I'm sure it did taste awful, but luckily had no adverse effects on him, although we did have to find out any potential reactions, as it had never been done before. Enema take two was administered and the procedure went ahead.

A well-known comedian attended for his colonoscopy and had us in absolute stitches throughout his procedure. Luckily, all was well, and a good day had by all.

Health promotion was a big part of the role and, in Bristol as opposed to Torbay, there were far more multicultural areas that did not access the programme. Therefore, we visited Somalian (and other ethnic minority) community hubs to explain the programmes. If we could alleviate concerns so that just one more person accessed the service, then it was worth it.

I loved my job. We worked across five sites, so it was never quiet, and I was back to scopes, visions of internal organs and it seemed like I had never been away. This time, although my role had changed, the procedure rooms felt very familiar. In my five or six years working in Bristol, I "acted up" to band seven, managing the team on two occasions; no one was more surprised than me about that. I loved it! The ability to have a voice in growing the service and advocating for the team, I was offered the permanent band seven, however it did not feel it was the right time for me to accept that as I was becoming more wistful of my previous life in the Bay. We had a lovely home and friends, but I missed living by the sea and, after many discussions and sleepless nights, we made a decision to move back to my beloved Torquay, where I now had a granddaughter I adored, and I looked forward to spending more time with family and friends.

I send off an email to the BCSP lead in Torbay, who I had known from the many years I had spent in endoscopy, to ask her to keep me in mind should something come up. I decided I wanted to drop my days to get more of a work-life balance and hoped I would be able to keep doing the job I loved.

After a few months, she did indeed contact me to tell me there would be a role coming up and I should apply. The house had an offer on it, but not finalised, however I also knew that this job may not come up again. So, after discussing it with Bob, I applied and got the role, starting in November 2019, so we rented a winter let for me for a few months whilst Bob stayed in Bristol to sell the house, and we went back to the old days of weekend get-togethers, apart from I had Barney, my lovely loyal dog, for company.

Although bowel screening is a national programme, each hub has its own way of working. There were some things done differently, but hopefully my experience and input would be useful and I soon settled into my new role. The team were great and very welcoming but on my first list I came face-to-face with the oh-so-impatient doctor from my OP clinic all those years ago.

I was more experienced and he had mellowed, so we got on just fine. A few months later, the sale of our home went through, and we bought our 'forever' home in Torbay. I felt settled and back where I belonged. My husband's (yes, by now he was my husband!) job was a bit more difficult from this area and he would have to travel a bit more, but had reconciled to it and life was good – and then everything changed.

In December 2019, it was reported there had been some people falling sick after visiting a seafood market in Wuhan and, by January 2020, it was reported that there was a virus spreading amongst people who had never visited the site, therefore certainty about human-to-human transmission was confirmed. It was subsequently named coronavirus (later shortened to Covid-19) caused by severe acute respiratory syndrome (SARS-CoV2). The first UK coronavirus case was reported in January and, by the end March 2020, 4,426 people had died. The World Health Organisation declared the outbreak a pandemic. At this time, my daughter was rushed to hospital to have an emergency caesarean at thirty-four weeks due to preeclampsia. I rushed up to Manchester where she was living and stayed for a few days, visiting her and my new grandson in hospital. He was in an incubator but doing well and she was dealing with it all so well, although it was a struggle to leave them both. As I came back to Torbay, I felt unwell, with chest tightness and a persistent cough, and was told to stay at home and self-isolate. There was no routine testing in place and I was just to assume I had Covid. The first lockdown was announced, non-essential businesses, schools, indoor sports venues and other activities all closed. People were advised to work from home if they could, children were being home schooled, we were told to practise social distancing and the NHS was beginning to feel the strain. At this time, members of my family became ill in Scotland with Covid and my niece (Maureen, who had so generously fundraised for me going to Cambodia) had the strain of her husband being admitted to ICU and intubated. He was in ICU for five weeks and in hospital for eight, he was desperately ill, but one of the lucky ones to come home. For me, workwise, nothing much changed. I continued to work but there was a slight decline in admissions; people with worsening conditions did not seek help, operations were cancelled and the economy was badly damaged. The nation was urged to 'clap for carers' on doorsteps every Thursday night to thank NHS workers for their role during the pandemic. In April 2020, I had a call from work on a Friday to say I was being redeployed to a Covid ward on the Monday, as cases had begun to rise again. It wasn't clear for how long, but our screening programme had been suspended, as had many areas of health, to focus on a rising number of Covid positive hospitalisations.

The last time I had worked on a ward was fourteen years before; I felt very anxious and concerned. And so,

I was back to being a ward nurse. The ward to which I was assigned had positive Covid patients and patients waiting on Covid test results. We were mask fitted and shown how to doff and don (basically getting all the gear on and off; masks, gloves, aprons, glasses), which had to be done every time you were in a room or bay with Covid confirmed patients. These were not the sickest of patients needing ventilation, as they moved to more intensive therapy wards or ICU, but they were sick, and we did have deaths. Every day, I went to work dreading what I would be facing. I had to familiarise myself with drug rounds again, complex intravenous medications, and the fear that I would do someone harm because of my lack of recent experience with very sick people was tangible. One of the worst things was speaking to relatives on the phone to tell them their loved one was dying. No visitors were allowed in but, in the cases where we had some awareness of close end of life, one family member could come in on one occasion. They had to have all the PPE on and then self-isolate when they went home for two weeks – not practical for most people – and sometimes we could only offer a call whilst we held a phone to the patient's ear. Listening to husbands, wives, sons, daughters, etc., telling their loved ones how much they loved them and crying, knowing they weren't going to see them again, was heartbreaking. There are no funny or light-hearted moments from my time on the ward. It was stressful, with not enough PPE, so the rules changed every day

– wear the mask for two hours, wear it for four now – new evidence or shortness of masks? Showering and changing before leaving for home every shift, but then eventually being told to take scrubs home to wash in my domestic washing machine because we didn't have enough and trying to allay the concerns of my husband whilst I was very concerned about taking any virus home. Whilst I initially felt proud that the nation was clapping and showing support, I became a little disillusioned with the government and their actions to protect us. I did this for six weeks, until our service was resumed, as it was then deemed as essential, as we may be missing potential cancers. Some of my nursing friends are still bravely working on these wards as I write this.

By June, it was thought that the worst of the pandemic was behind us, cases began to drop or plateau, and lockdown measures reduced or lifted. August saw 'eat out to help out' in which the government subsidised food and drink for three days a week and, whilst it may have helped the economy, I'm not sure it was the best use of public funding. By September, the virus was soaring again, and pharmaceutical companies were in a race to develop a vaccine.

I would often think about the lovely people I met in Cambodia and how on earth they would manage this global pandemic without vaccines, without masks, without the ability to distance or self-isolate. I firmly believed that the countries who had access to these vaccines needed to share with the ones who did not. The virus continued on, and a second lockdown took place in October 2020 with tier systems of restrictions in different areas of the country. The public were again urged to show their support by 'clapping for heroes', this time to support all the essential workers who carried on during the toughest times. Interestingly, a report in the *Nursing Times* said nurses did not want the clapping, they just wanted people to adhere to the rules and safety guidelines. They appreciated the good intentions, but they were tired and stressed whilst continuing to fight on; I understood that perfectly. On the 8th of December 2020, a lady in the UK became the first person in the world to be given an approved vaccine at her local hospital. The vaccine would make an impact, but not everyone would have it for whatever reasons. It was personal choice, which in this country would not become mandatory. At the time of writing this, there have been approximately 21.7 million cases in the UK and 171 thousand deaths.

And so, life went on and work continued, albeit with more restrictions and rules regarding PPE and the use of masks. I contracted Covid again in August 2021 and was quite poorly for a few days, losing my sense of taste and smell and generally feeling quite ill. I have been left with a change in my sense of smell and some muscle aches and pains.

In January 2022, I made a decision to bring my retirement forward a few months and spend more time enjoying the pleasures of life and family. I dip in and out now doing some bank shifts when staffing levels are low, but taking life more slowly, writing my book, crafting and smelling the roses (not the rosé) and I have just completed a holistic therapy course and plan to offer massage in my home spa room. Holistic therapies are very similar to nursing, looking at the whole person, realising the power of touch and caring. At this stage of life, I still feel I have something to offer, so yet another change of direction!

I have met some terrific people along the way, I have laughed and I have cried, I continued to have highs and lows, I met patients who touched my heart and some I would rather forget. I have had days where I felt like I couldn't carry on and that the NHS was floundering, but I did go on and I still believe in an NHS that is accessible to all. It's my NHS and your NHS and I am so proud to have been a part of it. Going forward, I think it needs an overhaul on how to fund it and a huge amount of education of the public to promote their own health and lifestyle choices. Despite its difficulties, how amazing that anyone, no matter how financially secure, can access healthcare, which is still free at the point of delivery, and based on clinical need and not the ability to pay. This was the belief of Aneurin Bevan on the 5th of July 1948 when the NHS was launched and it's a belief I still hold dear. We just need to find a way to retain it.

My book is a compilation of reflections of my

thoughts, feelings and experiences along my journey following my decision to change my life and career at the age of forty-eight. I realise it was brave and I have proven myself to be strong; I would not change a thing. To anyone who is contemplating change, it is never ever too late.

She believed she could,
so she did.

Acknowledgements

My thanks to Cassandra Welford who encouraged me to take up my pen again and finish my book.

To Jen Parker, Fuzzy Flamingo, for believing in my book and doing such a good job of encouraging me from the first time we spoke to the publishing of this book.

To Kimberley Reid-Fernandez for illustrating my book cover image and putting up with all my suggestions and changes.

To the Open University, an amazing establishment, pioneering learning and making it available to everyone. Without you I would not be where I am now.

To Rowcroft hospice who showed me a different way of nursing, a fantastic place full of inspirational people, staff and patients alike.

And lastly, but definitely not least, to Torbay and South Devon NHS Foundation Trust and the amazing colleagues, mentors and friends I have made over the years. Torbay Hospital supported me through four years of training and continued to support me as the Registered Nurse I became.

Printed in Great Britain
by Amazon

10717416R00106